A GUIDE TO POLARITY THERAPY:

THE GENTLE ART OF HANDS-ON HEALING

A GUIDE TO POLARITY THERAPY:

THE GENTLE ART OF HANDS-ON HEALING

Maruti Seidman

ELAN PRESS
BOULDER, COLORADO
1991

Editor—Douglas Menville
Cover/book design—Molly Gough
Illustrations—Sheryl McCartney and Nell Blackwell

First Edition May 1982
Revised, Enlarged Edition April 1986
Revised January 1991

This book is not intended to diagnose, prescribe or treat any ailment, nor is it in-tended in any way as a replacement for medical consultation when needed. The author and publishers of this book do not guarantee the efficacy of any of the treatments and techniques herein described, and strongly suggest that at the first suspicion of any disease or disorder, the reader consult a physician.

ELAN PRESS
Reprinted June 1995
9 8 7 6 5
Printed in the United States of America

Fear not the unknown
Pass through the waterfall of life
With love flowing from your heart.
Take nothing
But the immortality
Of your soul,
And light the skies,
Giving oneness to All.

       —Maruti

Polarity Balancing Certification Program

Maruti has been teaching and certifying practitioners since 1980. He is affiliated with many of the leading Massage Schools and Centers throughout the United States, where he teaches his basic 120 Hour Polarity Balancing Certification Program.

If you would like more information about his program and schedule, or want him to come to your community, please contact him at the address below.

Maruti Seidman
P.O. Box 3175
Boulder, Colorado 80307
or call toll free
1-800-334-4097

This book is dedicated
to my children, Daniel
and Alana.

ACKNOWLEDGMENTS

There are many people who gave much of their time and creative energy in helping me complete this book.

Dhyan Yogi guided me to a place of peace within.

Becky Sharman taught me how to be a teacher.

Pierre Pannetier shared his gentleness and wisdom.

Catherine Murray worked directly with me, editing, typing and supervising the layout.

Sheryl McCartney created all the charts and diagrams. Her work is inspirational and made my words come alive.

Others who helped with the typing, editing and layout of the first edition were: Sumati, Judi Siegel, Jeanne Thompson and Kathy Ornellas.

I would also like to thank all the wonderful people I worked with at Twin Lakes College of the Healing Arts, Santa Cruz.

Thanks to Michael T. Rasmussen and Johnson Publishing Company for making this edition possible.

To my sweetheart Sharada, for all her loving support.

Finally, I would like to thank all the people of this planet who are living their lives immersed in love.

The moment you notice
That you are just
An instrument of God,
The moment you become
Like a hollow flute,
The wind will blow through you
And there will be music.

—Dhyan Yogi

CONTENTS

Preface   ix
What Is Polarity Therapy?   1
Energy Currents   5
Modality in Polarity Therapy   9
Cultivating Trust and Non-Attachment   11
Preparation for Treatment   15
The Five Elements   17
The Ether Element   21
The Air Element   31
The Fire Element   43
The Water Element   47
The Earth Element   55
The Stomach   65
The Liver   69
The Kidneys   73
Diet   77
Chakra Balancing   87
The Five-Pointed Star   95
The Neck   97
The Chair Treatment   101
The Arms and Hands   105
The Hand Chart   109
The Back   113
The Hips   117
Perineal Session   119
Lengthening the Short Leg   123
Joint Session   127

The General Session. 131
Diagnostic Signs 133
Exercise 135
Pregnancy 141
About Fever. 147
Home and Herbal Remedies for Common Ailments 149
Quieting the Mind 155
The Polarity Love Circle 159
Songs to Open the Heart. 161
Bibliography. 165

LIST OF CHARTS

1. Elemental Relationship Between Fingers and Toes   7
2. The Skeletal System 19
3. The Organs. 20
4. Foot Chart: Reflexology and Acu-Points. 53
5. Summary of the Ayurvedic Theory of the Five Elements 63
6. Chakra Chart 89
7. Hand Chart. 108

PREFACE

The search for good health and longevity has been one of mankind's eternal preoccupations. True seekers find their answers only after looking deeply within their own beings.

This lengthy and difficult self-evaluation process is enough to deter most individuals. People do not want to look at, much less stir up, all their internal garbage. It is much easier to let things be! But for those of us who welcome the opportunity to recycle our fears, doubts and negativity, there are many wonderful proven systems available.

Polarity Therapy, created by Dr. Randolph Stone, is a holistic system enabling people to rediscover their inner beauty in a gentle way. Polarity promotes deep relaxation and revitalization by balancing the body's energy. Once you are relaxed, your own natural intelligence will automatically correct any temporary imbalance of energy, and good health will be restored.

Polarity works because it is designed to help the *whole* person, not just the part that hurts. Through love energy, positive thoughts and attitudes, gentle manipulations, mild exercise and proper dietary habits, a true feeling of wellness can be achieved.

Dr. Stone was a Doctor of Osteopathy and Naturopathy and a chiropractor. For over 60 years he helped people help themselves. He traveled around the world studying ancient healing techniques, including Acupuncture, Herbology, Eastern Massage, Foot Reflexology, Shiatsu Massage and Zone Therapy. Modern Polarity is a smooth blending of all this knowledge into a highly evolved system.

Dr. Stone passed on in December of 1981. He was 93 years old and spent his last ten years meditating at an ashram in India. Although I never had the pleasure of personally meeting Dr. Randolph Stone, I have touched upon his spirit through Polarity.

When Dr. Stone retired to India, he appointed Pierre Pannetier, N.D., his successor. Pierre continued the work Dr. Stone began, traveling across the U.S. giving Polarity seminars for the last 12 years. He recently passed on in the fall of 1984. I had the pleasure of studying with him and cherish the wisdom, gentleness and love he shared.

This book is a guide to Polarity Therapy for the beginner as well as the serious student. For more detailed information about polarity, I urge you to read all of Dr. Stone's books.

Maruti
P.O. Box 3175
Boulder, Colorado 80307

WHAT IS

POLARITY THERAPY?

Polarity Therapy seeks to harmonize people with their environment and nature. A healthy body is dependent on its ability to maintain free-flowing energy circuits. Any obstruction will result in pain and eventually illness. Acknowledging that our bodies consist of more than just skin, bones, organs, nerves and muscles is at the core of Polarity conceptualization. We *are* energy. All energy is governed by the three electromagnetic charges: positive, negative and neutral. Likewise, the entire body is viewed as an energy field with specific currents and patterns. These currents originally built the body and continue to operate until we leave it. When any one of these currents short-circuits, the entire energy field is affected. By understanding the relationships of the different currents and their charges we can proceed to balance them with our mind, body and spirit. Polarity Therapy is the science of balancing these subtle energy currents by using love, positive thoughts and attitudes, gentle manipulations, exercise and proper diet.

LOVE

Love energy connects our spirit to the Creator and has been described as the current of the soul. Love is something that everyone everywhere desires and we have difficulty existing without it. Love is everywhere: just look around and you'll see it being expressed. The flowers blooming in spring, a mother nursing her baby, people smiling or waving hello, a rainbow-colored sky are all expressions of love found every day throughout the world. Unfortunately for some, the quest for love has led them

1

to search high and low, round and round, without ever achieving their goal. Close your eyes and go within to see and feel your soul. It is here that love awaits you. It's been there all the time. You can't buy it at a store because it is given freely from one soul to another or from nature to us all.

Just as in life, Polarity Therapy centers around love energy. Our goal as practioners is to listen carefully to our clients' needs and allow them to feel secure enough to express themselves on whatever level necessary. Being compassionate and not judging your client's actions will enable the love to flow easily and clearly.

THOUGHTS AND ATTITUDES

Cultivating positive thought patterns is the key to health and happiness. When your thoughts are flowing freely, in harmony with Nature, there is peace and happiness. All tensions, energy blocks and sickness begin in the mind, then filter down and manifest in the body. Fear, negative thoughts, anxiety and stress create all sickness by stopping the flow of life-force energy within the body. As you eliminate negative thought patterns, you increase your physical and mental well-being. A healthy body is the reflection of a healthy mind. The two are inseparable. You are what you think.

You create your own reality and are responsible for your actions. Why become bound to negative thought patterns that can keep you off-balance and unhealthy? If you are sick or your life isn't manifesting as you planned, figure out why and regain control of your life. Too often you limit yourself by blaming other people for your own misfortune. This kind of thinking shows your confusion. It is up to you to re-program this negative thinking with positive thinking. Let the change be slow and easy. Be conscious of your thoughts, and the many obstacles the mind once created will slowly cease to exist. Your life will be easier, have more direction and purpose.

MANIPULATIONS

The object of the Polarity Therapy manipulations is to relax you, to allow your life currents to be brought into balance. When the life-force energy flows freely within the body, chronic blocks of tension that reside in the muscles, bones and internal organs disappear, allowing you to rediscover the sense of oneness that rests gently within all of us. The end result is the restoration of normal body and mind function.

EXERCISE

Like any complete exercise system, Polarity's easy stretching postures work on all parts of the body, increasing circulation and the elasticity of the muscles, bones and spine. The key Polarity stretching posture is the Squat Position, which is closely related to the position of the embryo in the mother's womb. This position attracts the five elements of Ether, Air, Fire, Water and Earth from the cosmic rays of life and is Nature's way of building a healthy body. Polarity exercises are easy to do and are appropriate for people of all ages.

DIET

There are no exact rules in discussing diet, because everyone is different. The best way to determine when to eat, how much to eat, what foods to eat at any meal, etc., is by trial and error. When you establish a strict code of rules for the consumption of food, you are limiting yourself. Any time you set limits, it stops your growth and creates blocks in your life-force energy. Enjoy your food, eat with love, try not to overeat, and eat the kinds of foods that bring balance and harmony.

ENERGY CURRENTS

Every manifestation of matter is regulated by the three electromagnetic fields of positive, negative and neutral. As these three electrical charges interact, they determine how matter functions. If there is an abundance of one charge or a lack of another, an imbalance occurs, affecting all three.

The planets revolving around the sun and the electrons and protons revolving around the nucleus of an atom are all expressions of matter in action. In human cells, positive energy is continuously moving *away* from the center, expanding outward on the right side. Negative energy is continuously moving *toward* the center, contracting downward on the left side. Both energies revolve around a central neutral axis.

This same relationship occurs in our bodies. The head and spinal column form the central neutral axis. The positive outward energy is expressed through the right side. The negative inward energy is expressed through the left side. The front of the body has a positive charge and the back has a negative charge. The top of the body has a positive charge, the middle section a neutral charge and the bottom a negative charge. Thus, the entire body is subdivided into different zones containing different electrical charges that all stem from the molecular manifestation of energy.

When an abundance of the outward, warm, positive energy current accumulates, a short-circuit, or blockage, occurs. This can result in pain and irritation. Using the opposite, or negative, charge is necessary to balance the overstimulated area. Simply place your left hand over the afflicted area and relief will come quickly. The currents are slowed, reduced, congested, contracted or spastic when there is too much inward negative energy constricting their flow. The remedy lies in the warmth and expanding energy represented by the right hand. Simply place it over the spasm for quick relief.

Since all Polarity contacts are bipolar, it is necessary to have both hands making contact on the body for best results. Position one hand over the inflamed or constricted area and the other on the opposite side. If the energy block is on the front of the body, place your left hand over the irritation and your right hand on the opposite contact of the back. If the energy block is on the back of the body, place your right hand over the spasm and your left hand on the opposite contact on the front. This double contact will draw the blocked energy through from the front to the back, or back to front, releasing the spasm or irritation. The same relationship holds true for side-to-side contacts as well as top-to-bottom contacts. As we do the manipulations with our hands, we are almost always in harmony with the energy currents—a positive charge is balancing a negative charge.

Remember: The *right side* represents warmth, heat, yang, the sun, positive, expanding energy. The *left side* represents cooling, contracting, yin, the moon, negative, receptive, inward energy.

THE BODY'S CURRENTS

There are five major currents in the body. The first is the *core current* of the torso that flows from north to south, or from the head to the pelvis, then up the back to the head again. This current represents the Ether Element. The second one runs from east to west, from the front to the back in a circular pattern, and is called the *surface lateral current*. It is like a vortex and covers the entire body from head to foot. This current represents the Air Element. Third is the *diagonal current* that is found on both sides of the body; it starts at the shoulders and goes to the opposite hips along diagonal lines. It is part of the figure-eight pattern found throughout the entire body. This current represents the Fire Element. Fourth is the *long current* that splits the body in half; it extends from the head to the foot, including the arms and hands. On the right side it moves in a clockwise motion; on the left side in a counter-clockwise motion. This current represents the Water Element. Fifth is the current that zig-zags in solid *straight lines* from one side of the body to the other. This current represents the Earth Element. The fingers and toes also have both a charge and an elemental relationship (see chart 1). The thumb represents the Ether Element and has a neutral charge. The index finger represents the Air Element and has a negative charge. The middle finger represents the Fire Element and has a positive charge. The ring finger represents the Water Element and has a negative charge. The little finger represents the Earth Element and has a positive charge. The same holds true for the toes,

THE ELEMENTAL RELATIONSHIP
BETWEEN THE FINGERS & TOES

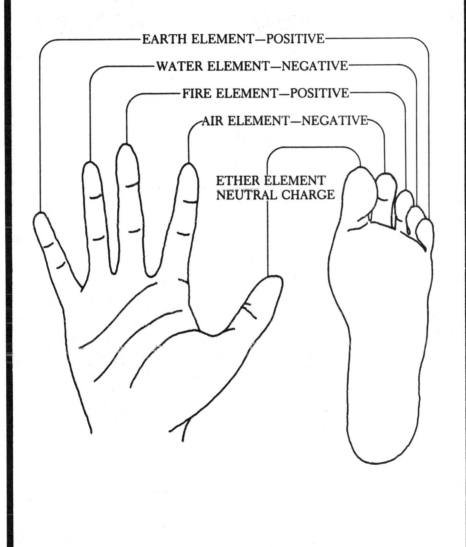

EARTH ELEMENT—POSITIVE

WATER ELEMENT—NEGATIVE

FIRE ELEMENT—POSITIVE

AIR ELEMENT—NEGATIVE

ETHER ELEMENT
NEUTRAL CHARGE

with the big toe equal to the thumb and the little toe equal to the little finger. The other toes correspond to their opposite fingers.

ENERGY BLOCKS

Chronic energy blocks are most frequently the result of an accumulation of energy at the negative electrical pole. The blocked energy must be persuaded to flow outward from within. Once the negative pole has been released, activating the positively charged pole of that energy circuit will restore proper function.

Too often we only look at the physical body when pain and disease occur. The body receives all the blame without our realizing that the disease process originates in the mind. People who lack the motivation and desire to consciously alter their negative mental processes will never really respond to therapy. At best, their relief will be temporary. Many people enjoy the extra attention received from friends and relatives while being sick. It may be the only time they receive love and understanding, and they don't want to give it up. Sometimes it takes a life-threatening situation like a heart attack, stroke or confirmation of cancer before people receive sufficient motivation to change their lifestyle, diet and thinking process. And even then, some find many excuses to continue living the same destructive way, hoping an operation or a miracle pill will cure them.

Don't make the mistake of getting upset at people who come to you for treatment and advice and then are slow to change. Everyone changes at their own pace and the best you can do is love them regardless of what they do or don't do. The more you can give gentle guidance and treatments and channel love, the better off everyone will be. Asking or demanding that people drastically change everything about themselves in a short period of time is not realistic. Let the change be slow and easy, so that they can cultivate a new lifestyle at a pace that suits them.

MODALITY IN POLARITY THERAPY

There are three basic ways to touch a body while giving a treatment: *gently*, *actively* and *deeply*, and each has its own special effect. When you touch someone in a *gentle* way, it brings about deep relaxation by calming the nervous system. Everyone responds well to the gentle touch. For some, it may be the only time they receive any tenderness in their lives. When you touch someone in an *active* way, there is always movement, such as rocking. This has a tendency to stir things up and is wonderful for people who need to be stimulated. The individual who has poor circulation or digestion responds well and enjoys the active touch, as it gets their energy moving. When you touch someone *deeply*, it usually brings about intense pain and causes a quick detoxification within the system. Some people are under the impression that without pain, there's no gain. This might be true for some of the bodywork systems that use the deep touch; however, in Polarity Therapy we have come to the conclusion that using deeply applied force to the muscles, bones and internal organs only causes people to tighten up as they unconsciously defend themselves against the invasion of their body. If you are trying to help people relax, it doesn't make sense to use a deep touch that causes them to tighten up.

There is an electrical field around every living thing called an *aura*. From your fingertips, your aura extends out about six to ten inches. When your hands touch another person, your aura is strong enough to go completely through most parts of the body. With this in mind, it is unnecessary to touch anyone deeply, because the auric extension of your energy field can do the work gently, safely and effectively.

CULTIVATING TRUST AND

NON-ATTACHMENT

When a person gets on your table for a treatment they are placing themselves in your hands. Sometimes the most difficult part of the threatment for your client is to allow you to touch them. Hands-on healing is an intimate experience for both the practitioner and the client, demanding a certain amount of trust between both individuals for it to be successful. You might be the best practitioner in your area with the most advanced techniques and a fine reputation, but what good does all that do if when you meet your new clients, they don't feel comfortable around you? Regardless of the style of hands-on healing you have been trained in, the most important aspect of your treatments is how well your clients respond to you as a person. If your clients like you, feel comfortable around you and enjoy spending time with you, then your treatments with them will be positive and successful. If your clients trust you, they will be more apt to let go of their energy blocks during the treatment because they feel safe.

Cultivating people's trust depends largely on your relationship with yourself. If you are happy, enjoy life, trust your intuition, have a relationship with God, are easy going and have a strong desire to help your fellow man or woman, then your potential clients will immediately pick up on your vibrations and good intentions and feel at ease around you. If your life is in order and you are at peace with yourself, your clients will feel that peace and trust you. It is important to send out lots of love when you first meet your potential clients. Talk with them in an easy manner, be honest, listen to what they say and tell them about yourself and your background. Tell them what kind of treatments you do and what they can expect from them. Mention how long the treatment will last, whether it will hurt them or not, what parts of their bodies you will be touching and what effects the treatment will have on them.

NON-ATTACHMENT

We must ask ourselves: are we healers? Do we really heal people who come to us for treatments? The answer is no. People heal themselves. When you place too much emphasis on the outcome of a treatment, your ability to be a clear channel for the love energy is blocked. When desired results are not obtained, you may blame yourself because you thought you were doing the healing. When you cultivate non-attachment, the channel opens and the love energy flows freely like a newly formed mountain stream. Always remember that your job is to help facilitate the healing process and help empower people to heal themselves.

When people realize that they alone must take responsibility for their health and that they can control their own destiny, they can begin their healing journey. When their fear subsides, the white light of God will shine through them, illuminating their minds. As a friend and practitioner you must focus on the love energy, and the results of the treatments will take care of themselves. If at first you have difficulty being unattached, don't get discouraged. The more treatments you do, the easier it gets, and you'll learn to trust yourself more and more.

TENDER SPOTS

Just as a stream can become blocked and stagnate, so can the flow of energy in your body become blocked and cause a tender spot. As your bodywork career progresses you'll notice that every body is different in shape, structure and resistance to your touch. The level of pressure you can use effectively on one person will make another jump right off the table. As you work with your client, get constant feedback on how they are feeling. When you discover tender spots it's best to have your client start a series of deep breaths while you apply pressure to gently work out those spots. A pattern of slow, deep inhalations and exhalations works best. The breathing will take your client's mind off the pain and allow them to feel relaxed. The major releases will occur when they exhale, so you can work a little more actively then (if they give you permission), thus promoting more cleansing. You will be amazed at how easily and quickly painful spots will become unblocked.

The more releases, the better off your clients are. If people don't want to let go, be patient. After you get to know them and they trust you more, they'll feel secure and relaxed enough to release the blocked energy and re-establish the energy flow. If you try to force a deep release, even though you think they need it, many problems can arise.

I once attended a class in which the instructor tried to break through a student's chronic shoulder pain while demonstrating a treatment in class. She was not ready to let it go and resisted the instructor's treatment. The end result was that the woman never released her tension and the instructor never let up. Both were in tears by the end of the treatment. The student was in great pain (just the opposite of what a Polarity treatment is all about) and the instructor realized he had made a mistake. The lesson is: Don't let your ego get in the way of your treatments, don't ever use force during a treatment and don't be attached to the results of the treatment. Just do the work and whatever is supposed to happen, will.

PULSE READING

Pulse reading is an art form used to help you get a better idea of what is actually going on within your client's body. Sometimes it is difficult to get an accurate response when you ask your client how they are doing. Most of the time, people are unaware of what's happening with their own health and are unable to answer that question accurately. The pulses don't lie: they represent a highly evolved system of determining how the body is functioning.

Pulse reading has evolved through the centuries in accordance with different schools of thought, each perfecting its own way. I don't think any one system is better than the other, as they are all aimed at accomplishing the same results—good health and longevity. For our purposes, we will use the pulses located on the sides of the neck (carotid artery), and at the *flexor longus*, below the inside ankle bones in the feet. By feeling the pulses' strength and rate of beat, you can determine if there is any imbalance in the body elements, and thus design your session specifically to harmonize the imbalanced elements. At first it may seem difficult to feel the pulses; however, with practice you can develop your sensitivity and learn to distinguish the pulses accurately.

If the pulse is weak and you can hardly feel it, the *Water Element* is out of balance. If the pulses have the same strength, but vary in cadence from left to right (in a zig-zag pattern), the *Air Element* is out of balance. If one of the pulses is strong and the other ones are weak, the *Fire Element* is out of balance. A healthy pulse is strong, symmetrical and has a clear cadence.

Pulse reading is a delicate art that requires practice, awareness in your fingertips, and a willingness to serve others. *Ayurveda,* an ancient Indian healing system, describes over a hundred pulses, which take at least 20 years to master. The above describes the three main pulses.

PREPARATION FOR

TREATMENT

In preparation for any treatment, I follow a certain well-balanced guideline. My first consideration is where the session will take place. Ideally, a room that is quiet, clean and well-ventilated is recommended. This may be a special room in your home, a rented room in a spa or some other relaxed location. However, if no such place exists for you, don't worry, anywhere in your home will be all right. I have given many treatments on a foam pad on the floor in my living room with wonderful results. Be flexible enough to adjust to any circumstances you are faced with.

My next concern is with myself: How am I feeling? Am I alert, centered and ready, or do I feel spacey, off center or unsure of myself? If you are not ready to give a treatment, there are many things you can do to bring yourself back to your own peace within. The easiest way to regroup your energy is through meditation: sitting quietly and watching all the mind's thoughts flash by will eventually lead you to a point of stillness that is refreshing and regenerating. If you have trouble sitting quietly in meditation, try a few minutes of exercise. Exercising will bring new blood running through your system and can break through any blocked energy you may have. Hatha Yoga, Tai-Chi, or any creative movement system are all fine and achieve the same results.

Sometimes practitioners complain of picking up negative energy or actual sickness from their clients while doing a treatment. Pierre Pannetier, the world's foremost authority on Polarity, says this occurs because we try too hard to help our clients and in doing so are really using force instead of love. When we use force we limit ourselves, creating unnecessary difficulties. Remember, it is not you who heals anyone; people heal themselves. You are just the catalyst in their healing process. So be unattached to the results of your treatment, and let the energy do the work!

Another way to prevent yourself from receiving any unwanted energy is to envision yourself surrounded by a bubble of white light. Saying a prayer to God for guidance before any treatment will also keep you centered. If none of this works, visualize your client's energy passing through you and going ten miles down into the earth during your treatment. The earth will gladly take any excess energy. Throughout the treatment, shake off excess energy from your hands to the floor, and immediately after the treatment wash your hands in cold water. Again, this will help you stay unaffected by your client's energy. Above all, trust yourself and don't be fearful of absorbing the ailments of your client.

POSITIONING FOR MANIPULATIONS

The bodywork technique described throughout this book will constantly refer to positioning yourself at various locations around the table your client is lying on. All the different positions will revolve around the main starting point, which is facing the head of your client on the table. Always move to your right or left when indicated; don't be concerned with the right or left side of your client when determining your position. Understanding this will guide you to the right position every time.

THE BODYWORK TABLE

It's very important to give your treatments on a table that is well suited for you. If you're working on a table that is either too high or too low, your body will probably feel it when your treatment is completed. If you strain yourself while giving treatments, you'll be defeating yourself. Ideally, the top of your table should not be any higher than the palms of your hands when they are brought to a parallel position to the floor as you stand with your hands by your side. Any variation from this height will probably cause you to strain while giving your treatment.

Your table should be constructed so that it doesn't make any noise as it rocks during the treatment. Nothing can be more distracting than a squeaking table. Make sure your table can support the weight of large people. Having a table collapse during a treatment is something you want to avoid. Open and close the table to see how difficult it is to assemble. Make sure the table is not too heavy to carry around. Buy your table from someone you know, or someone with a strong recommendation from a close friend. There are many people making tables today with new and unproven designs, so test it out thoroughly before you purchase it. A new table should cost from $200 to $400, depending on the manufacturer and the guarantee.

THE FIVE ELEMENTS

The elemental system of Ether, Air, Fire, Water and Earth is derived from ancient systems of holistic healing that originated in the East. Over five thousand years old, the concept of holistic medicine—balancing body, mind and spirit as one—has only recently gained some acceptance in the West, where for centuries physicians have based their work on the western system of thought originated by Aristotle. He developed the idea of the four elements—Air, Fire, Water and Earth—from which was derived the western medieval theory of the "four humours" of the body. The West gradually abandoned the concept of holistic medicine in favor of the scientific approach, but the East still practices it today, little changed from its origins in antiquity. Both systems have value, as the West is only now beginning to understand.

The holistic system adds a fifth element to the others—Ether, an extremely subtle, esoteric element from which the other four, more denser, elements manifested. Since the five elements play an important role in understanding Polarity Therapy, it's essential that we have a clear idea of what these elements are, where they are located in terms of the body, and how to balance them properly within ourselves.

The philosophical foundation supporting the eastern system of holistic medicine is perhaps best described by Dr. Vasant Lad in his excellent book, *Ayurveda: The Science of Self Healing*. According to Dr. Lad, the universe originally existed in a formless state of pure consciousness. A subtle vibration spontaneously arose from that formlessness to become the cosmic sound OM. The Ether Element originated from that sound and became the vehicle through which the other elements appeared. To this day the Ether Element is still the direct link to cosmic consciousness, and it is this fundamental relationship between man and the ethers that ultimately de-

---

termines his state of balance or imbalance with his environment and his soul.

As the Ether Element was set in motion, the Air Element was created. The motion of the Air Element created heat and light, forming the Fire Element. The Water Element was created as the heat of the Fire Element liquified parts of the melted ethers. When the Water Element crystallized it formed the Earth Element. Thus, the five elements of Ether, Air, Fire, Water and Earth came to be.

The five elements are present in all things. We can see this relationship clearly by examining water. When water has crystallized into ice, it is representative of the Earth Element. The Fire Element manifesting as heat melts the ice, which becomes water. When water boils and turns to steam, it reflects the Air Element. As the steam evaporates into space, it becomes part of the Ether Element. By saying that man is a microcosm of the macrocosm we are expressing man's fundamental relationship with the universe. We can't separate one from the other. Cosmic consciousness created the five elements, which are contained in all animate and inanimate things.

All matter is represented in the form of the five elements. They function throughout the body as a positive, negative or neutral electromagnetic response to external and internal stimuli. A miniature zodiac of 12 centers (the four elements of Air, Fire, Water and Earth times the three electromagnetic charges) is created within the body, linking man to the universe. This relationship with nature enables man to attract the finer energy patterns from the cosmos which then build, repair and maintain his form on this planet. This concept is often overlooked because it functions so quietly.

Did you ever notice how good it feels to assume the fetal position, especially when you're tired or sick? Ever wonder why? You spent the first part of your life growing in your mother's womb, secure in the fetal position of legs pointed upward toward the head and arms folded across the chest. The five elements of Ether, Air, Fire, Water and Earth are attracted to the fetus because all its electromagnetic poles are close to each other. This enables the fetus to respond quickly to all stimuli, resulting in rapid growth. Although you are no longer a fetus, assuming the fetal position reunites you with the five elements in the same way. Thus your energy currents can function more effectively, enabling you to feel calm and balanced.

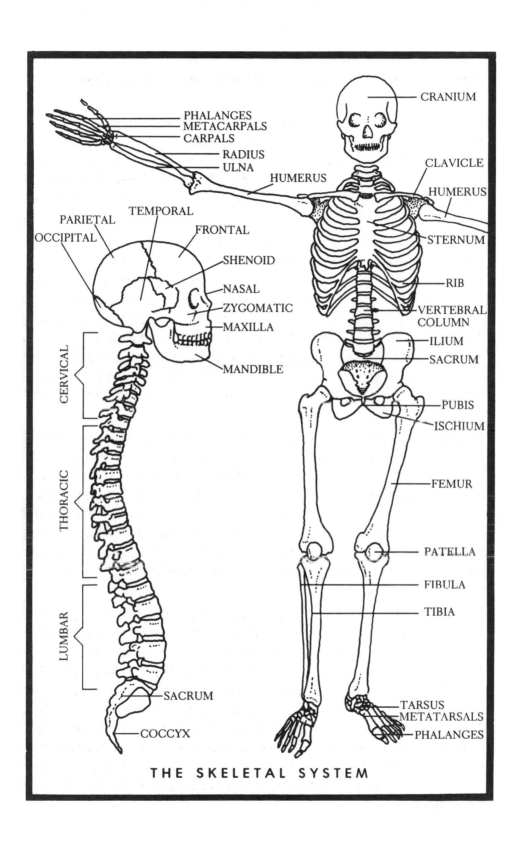

PHALANGES
METACARPALS
CARPALS
RADIUS
ULNA
HUMERUS
CRANIUM
CLAVICLE
HUMERUS
STERNUM
RIB
VERTEBRAL COLUMN
ILIUM
SACRUM
PUBIS
ISCHIUM
FEMUR
PATELLA
FIBULA
TIBIA
TARSUS
METATARSALS
PHALANGES

PARIETAL
OCCIPITAL
TEMPORAL
FRONTAL
SHENOID
NASAL
ZYGOMATIC
MAXILLA
MANDIBLE

CERVICAL
THORACIC
LUMBAR

SACRUM
COCCYX

THE SKELETAL SYSTEM

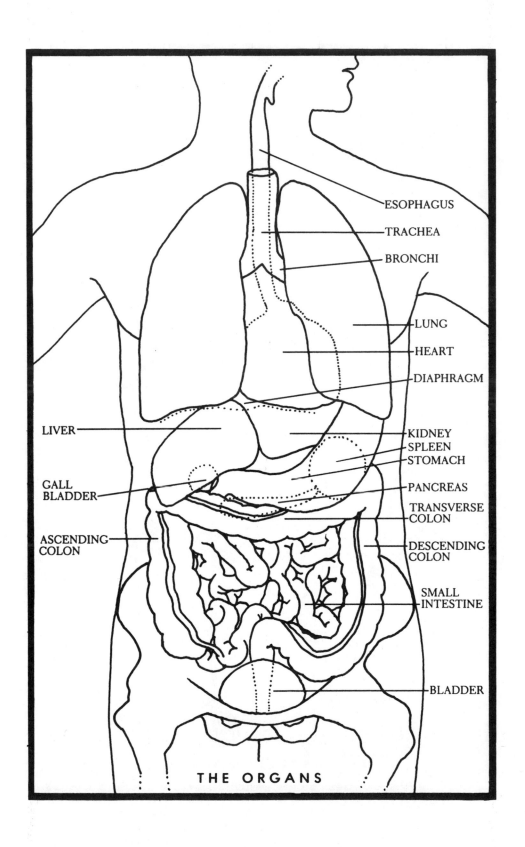

ESOPHAGUS

TRACHEA

BRONCHI

LUNG

HEART

DIAPHRAGM

LIVER

KIDNEY
SPLEEN
STOMACH

GALL
BLADDER

PANCREAS

TRANSVERSE
COLON

ASCENDING
COLON

DESCENDING
COLON

SMALL
INTESTINE

BLADDER

THE ORGANS

THE ETHER ELEMENT

The etheric energy pattern is the neutral force that flows continuously from the depths of the universe, linking man to the Creator. All physical manifestations of matter originate from the ethers. In the human body all the hollow spaces, including the center of the spinal column, the veins, arteries, nerves, internal organs and different body cavities, represent the Ether Element. It is the subtlest of all the elements and its vibration is a representation of divine energy. The three electrical poles of the body associated with the Ether Element are the head (positive pole), the sacrum (neutral pole) and the arch of the foot (negative pole).

When the Ether Element combines with the other elements, certain qualities are manifested. The quality of nothingness is the dominating characteristic of the Ether Element. When the Ether Element combines with the Air Element, desire is formed. When the Ether Element combines with the Fire Element, anger is formed. When the Ether Element combines with the Water Element, attachment is formed. When the Ether Element combines with the Earth Element, fear is formed.

When we work with the head and spinal column, it's extremely important to be very gentle. The Ether Element represents a pure vibration and responds to gentleness and love. Any deep pressure applied to the head or spinal column can cause damage to the brain and nervous system, so never work deeply there. This treatment will allow your client to relax deeply and possibly go into a meditative state. This can help the person gain insight into why they are manifesting energy blocks in different parts of their body. Often people come back refreshed and ready to go. Sometimes people have flashes of old unresolved experiences which they have suppressed for many years. This is a good time for them to face these old traumas and let them go. Anyone suffering from exhaustion, nervous tension, anxiety, stress, headaches, irritability or confusion will greatly benefit from this treatment. Even if they don't have any major symptoms of disease, the deep relaxation they receive will allow them to feel peaceful again.

THE NERVOUS SYSTEM

Since this treatment centers around the head, spinal column and nervous system, understanding their relationship to the body will be helpful. The nervous system oversees all communications throughout the body. Its two main objectives are to induce movement and to work with the endocrine system to ensure balance and harmony between the body and its environment (homeostasis). The endocrine system secretes into the blood hormones that regulate certain activities of the body. Some of these hormones are either stimulated or inhibited by the nervous system; likewise, they can stimulate or inhibit the nerve impulses. Thus, both systems work together for the betterment of the whole unit. All the systems of the body function via nerve impulses. The nervous system judges how you are relating to your environment and then signals for any adjustment necessary to maintain equilibrium. For example, if you get into a "flight-or-fight" situation, the nerve impulses stimulate the endocrine system to secrete the hormone adrenaline, which gives you the energy to retreat quickly or stand your ground and battle it out. If you're walking down the street and you see someone pinned under a car, the same process may give you the strength to help move the car off the person. Under ordinary circumstances you probably wouldn't have the energy to accomplish such a feat.

COMPONENTS OF THE NERVOUS SYSTEM

The two main components of the nervous system are the *central nervous system* and the *peripheral nervous system*. The brain and spinal cord comprise the central nervous system, which interprets all incoming and outgoing sensations and impulses. The peripheral nervous system is comprised of *neurons* that link the brain and spinal cord to the glands, muscles and sensory receptors. The peripheral nervous system is subdivided into the *afferent* and *efferent* systems. The afferent system relays messages from the outside of the body to the central nervous system, via the sensory neurons. The sensory neurons let the central nervous system know what's happening in the environment. The efferent system is comprised of nerve cells called *motor neurons,* which carry messages from the central nervous system to all the glands and muscles.

The efferent system is further divided into the *somatic nervous system* and the *autonomic nervous system*. The somatic nervous system communicates impulses from the central nervous system to the skeletal muscles and is therefore considered to transmit *voluntary* acts.

The autonomic nervous system is said to be *involuntary* because it sends impulses from the central nervous system to the smooth muscle tissue, cardiac muscle tissue and the glands, which function by themselves, unconsciously. The autonomic nervous system is comprised of the *sympathetic* and *parasympathetic* nervous systems. The sympathetic nervous system is responsible for the body's reaction in a flight-or-fight situation by speeding up the heart rate, raising the blood pressure and dilating the pupils of the eyes. It reacts when the body must put out energy. The parasympathetic nervous system functions when the body is resting and rejuvenating its lost energy supply. During digestion and absorption, when the body is breaking down its fuel for energy, the parasympathetic nervous system is working.

THE BRAIN

The brain is a mushroom-shaped organ that is a continuation of the spinal column. It is divided into four major parts: the *cerebrum, cerebellum, medulla oblongata* and *diecepholom*. The medulla oblongata attaches to the spinal column and is also called the *brain stem*. The cerebellum lies behind the brain stem and below the cerebrum. The diecepholom consists of the *thalamus* and the *hypothalamus* and is located above the brain stem. The cerebrum is the largest part of the brain, filling up most of the skull. The brain is protected by the hard cranial bones of the skull, with a few layers of *meninges* (membranes) surrounding it to prevent friction.

The brain is the body's main computer: it sends and receives messages via electrical impulses throughout the body. All bodily functions, including eating, sleeping, pain, muscular movement, etc., are controlled by the brain.

THE SPINAL COLUMN

The spinal column extends from the medulla oblongata, the base of the brain, down to the *ilium*, or hip area. It is comprised of five sections, totaling 33 vertebrae. There are seven vertebrae in the neck called *cervical*, 12 in the upper and mid-back called *thoracic*, five in the lower back called *lumbar*, five (fused together in adulthood) where the spinal column meets the hips called *sacral* and four (fused together in adulthood) extending down to form the tail bone, or *coccyx*. Each vertebra, with the exception of the *atlas* and the *axis* (the first and second), is comprised of a *vertebral body* and *arch*. Between each vertebral body is a vertebral *disc* that absorbs shock. The vertebral arch creates an open space called the *vertebral foramen* and the spinal column extends through the arch.

Muscles, ligaments and ribs attach to the spinal column at the *spinous process* and the two *transverse processes*, which are extensions of the vertebral arch. Each vertebral arch merges with the one next to it to form a ball-and-socket joint. These ball-and-socket joints neutralize the friction that occurs as the vertebrae move.

There are 31 pairs of spinal nerves that extend from the spinal column which transfer sensory impulses from the peripheral nervous system to the brain and motor impulses from the brain to the peripheral nervous system.

TECHNIQUE TO BALANCE THE ETHER ELEMENT

Remember, all contacts are light and soothing to the touch and are generally symmetrical. All holds should be sustained for at least three to five minutes, longer if you have the time. Make sure you are centered before you touch anyone. Squat and talk with your client beforehand and find out what is going on in their life—how their digestion and elimination are, if there has been any stress recently, or whatever else might be happening with them. The more you can get your client to participate and take responsibility for themselves, the more effective your session will be.

1. Halo

Have your client lie down on the table on their back. With palms open and fingers together, place both hands facing each other about three to four inches from your client's ears. This will let you enter their aura and unite with their energy in a soft, loving way.

2. Face Element Balancing

Place your earth finger just above the end of your client's eyebrow. Let your other fingers fall into place along the forehead (above the eyebrow) so that your air finger is just above the nose and your thumbs are along the crown of the head.

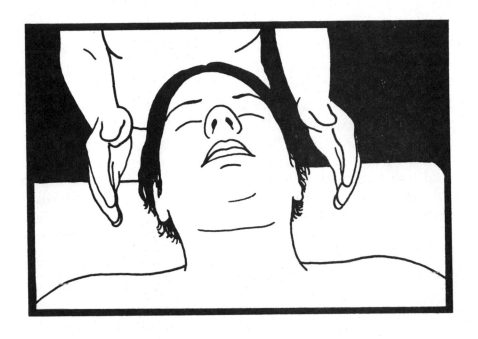

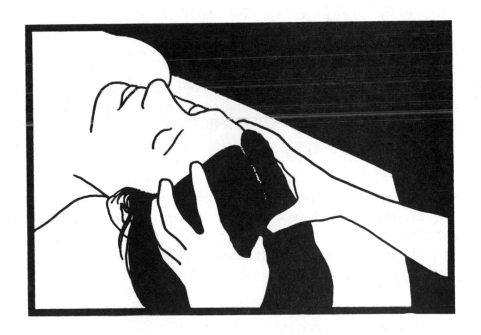

3. Skull Traction

Pick up your client's head with your left hand. Then gently place your right hand horizontally under the client's head, along the *occipital ridge* (at the back of the skull). Now place your left hand back on the forehead horizontally and hold. This is also good for emotional stress and can ease a pounding headache.

4. Head Cradle

Spread your fingers apart so that the ether and air fingers are together and the fire, water and earth fingers are together. Overlap your hands (the left under the right) under the occipital ridge and place your air fingers alongside the *vegas nerves* that run down the neck. Place your thumbs by the air fingers, under the ears. This brings into balance the parasympathetic nervous system, which deals with all involuntary actions.

5. Forgetting Cradle

Place your right hand under your client's head, with the occipital ridge resting between the ether and air fingers. Then, place your left hand on the forehead, with the fire and water fingers at the *third eye* (above and between the eyes), the earth and air fingers on the ridge above the eyebrows and the ether fingers on the *fontanel* (the top of the skull). This cradle will quiet a person's mind and calm their emotions.

6. Third Eye-to-Umbilicus Hold

Move to the right side of the table. Gently place your left hand on your client's forehead and your right hand on their navel. This will be good for all digestion difficulties and will revitalize the currents of the torso.

7. Element Balancing of the Toes

Move down to the feet. Gently place the thumb of your inside hand below your client's ankle bone. With the air fingertip of your outside hand, touch the toe tips gently, starting with the earth toe and moving up to the big toe. This is very soothing at the end of a session. There will be many releases of different degrees throughout the body while you are doing this manipulation.

TECHNIQUES TO BALANCE THE ETHER ELEMENT VIA THE NERVOUS SYSTEM

These manipulations are designed to balance the sympathetic and parasympathetic nervous systems. A sense of deep relaxation and tranquility will be experienced by anyone who receives this treatment. In today's world the calm, serene person is rare. As a group of people we seem to be obsessed with a fast-paced, intense lifestyle that places our bodies and minds under constant stress. This treatment will counteract the accumulated stress by reuniting the energy pattern of the nervous system. For the sympathetic nervous system the occipital ridge is the positive pole, the sacrum is the neutral pole and the heel is the negative pole. When there are too many impulses flowing downward, they produce breaks in the current below. When there are breaks in the circuit below due to trauma, the current above also suffers. The top affects the bottom and vice versa. When you find tension in one area, its opposite counterpart must also be worked on or your effort will be nothing more than a bandaid.

TECHNIQUE FOR THE SYMPATHETIC NERVOUS SYSTEM

The Occiput-to-Sacrum Hold is applied to both sides of the body, so it doesn't matter which side you begin on. Have your client lie on their stomach. Stand on the left side of the table; with your upper air finger, find a sore spot on the left occipital ridge. Place the fire finger of your lower hand on top of the right side of the sacrum (hip bone). Hold for three minutes. Release and repeat the hold on the other side. Now you

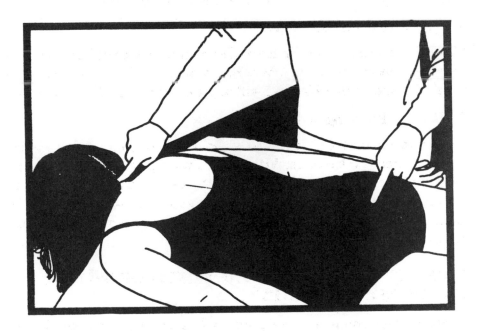

should be on the right side of the table. Place the air finger of your upper hand on the bottom of the left side of the sacrum and the ether and air fingers of your lower hand on the achilles tendon (heel) of the foot. Hold for three minutes. Repeat the hold on the other side.

TECHNIQUE FOR THE PARASYMPATHETIC NERVOUS SYSTEM

The Buttocks-to-Shoulder Contact begins as you stand to the right of your client. Place your left air finger on the end of the opposite shoulder and your right fire finger on the outside crease of the buttocks near the *femur* (thigh bone) of the leg closest to you. Hold for one to two minutes. Now move the left-hand contact to the mid-shoulder and the right-hand contact to the mid-crease of the buttocks. Hold for one to two minutes. Now

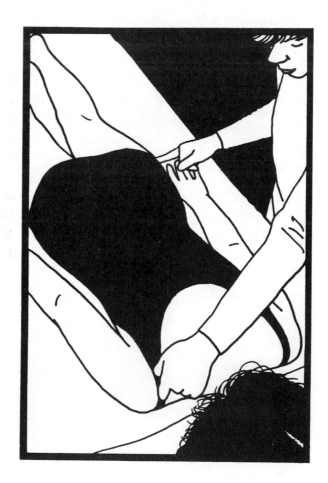

move your left-hand contact to where the shoulder meets the neck and your right-hand contact to where the crease meets the inside thigh. Hold for one to two minutes. Repeat this series of holds on the other side. This will induce a state of extreme relaxation. I have used this technique many times with wonderful results.

GETTING OFF THE TABLE

It's very easy for people to strain themselves while getting off the table. If this occurs, all the good you did during the session will be of no value. Most people will want to sit up after a session, straining their back or stomach. Quite often, many people will be so relaxed after a session that it will be difficult for them to move. The proper way for your client to get up is for them to roll over to either side. Then have them place their hands, palms down, on the table by their upper body and slowly push up to a sitting position. They will then be upright and feeling well.

BRUSHING OFF

At this point it is extremely important to brush off your client. After a treatment, there is a great deal of excess energy still surrounding them; it is in their aura and if not brushed off properly will resettle back down upon them. By brushing off your client, this can be avoided. Stand behind your client and place your right hand off their right shoulder about three inches and your left hand off their left shoulder about three inches. Now criss-cross your hands so that they are on opposite shoulders; continue this process, going down the back, criss-crossing three times. Once at the hips, drain off the energy into the ground. Now go to the front and brush straight down the torso and legs to the floor. Repeat the process of brushing off both the front and back three times.

THE AIR ELEMENT

The Air Element represents the respiratory and circulatory systems. The organs governed by the Air Element are the heart, the center of circulation, and the lungs, the center of respiration. The heart pumps the blood to all tissues. The lungs draw in energy from the air and filter the air from outside to provide oxygen to the blood.

Nothing can live without air. It is the sustaining energy in life that supplies the system with oxygen, which is essential for proper oxidation and combustion in the blood stream. Without enough air, the blood becomes sluggish, resulting in deposits of unused materials in the body's tissues. The three poles of the Air Element in the body are: Gemini, the shoulders, the positive pole, which rules the symmetry of the body and the balance between the two sides; Libra, the kidneys, the neutral pole; and Aquarius, the ankles, the negative. When the Air Element combines with the other elements, certain qualities are manifested. Speed is the dominating characteristic of the Air Element. When the Air Element combines with the Ether Element, the quality of lengthening is created. When the Air Element combines with the Fire Element, shaking is created. When the Air Element combines with the Water Element, movement is created. When the Air Element combines with the Earth Element, contraction is created.

As the Air Element comes into balance, one feels calm and relaxed. Most nervous and emotional tensions disappear and a sense of well-being prevails. The Air contacts affect the lateral surface currents (east to west), which rule the sense of touch in the skin. These currents are constantly telling the body what is going on in relation to its environment. There are many foods that fall under the classification of "airy," such as acidic fruits, nuts, fermented dairy products, yeast, apples and tomatoes. Foods that contain the Air Element are sour in taste and when consumed in moderation are beneficial. However, when too many of these foods are consumed they sour in the system, causing fermentation and gas. If this gas doesn't escape, it is stored in the muscles, ligaments and bones, causing many problems.

A detailed look at the heart and lungs will give us a better understanding of how the Air Element works within the body.

THE LUNGS

The lungs are two sponge-like sacks located in the *thoracic cavity* (chest), separated by the heart. They lie just below the *clavicles* (collar bones), above the *diaphragm* (a muscle that helps you breathe) and directly against the ribs in the front and back. The lungs are protected by two layers of membranes: one layer holds them in place and the other protects them from the ribs. In between these layers is a fluid that lubricates the membranes and prevents friction during breathing.

As the diaphragm contracts, the lungs fill up with fresh air. The heart pumps used blood into the lungs, where it deposits carbon dioxide and receives new oxygen in return. Then the blood is returned to the heart and pumped throughout the body via the arteries. When the diaphragm relaxes, carbon dioxide is exhaled from the body. The body can't survive without a constant fresh supply of oxygen, which is needed for oxidation to occur in the blood. Without proper oxidation, the body's nutrients can't be used economically. This results in the blood being filled with waste products, making it sluggish. If the blood remains sluggish, a loss of vitality is inevitable. Every cell in the body needs oxygen in order to perform its task; the brain needs a large supply of oxygen just to survive. It uses about 25 percent of the body's oxygen supply for its daily needs. Mental work can be more fatiguing than physical work because there is rarely any increased breathing rate or oxygen intake while you are sitting down and concentrating. However, in physical work the heart rate and breathing rate are dramatically increased, resulting in fresh, oxygenated blood being delivered throughout the system.

THE HEART

The heart lies between the lungs in the center of the chest cavity. About 67 percent of the heart lies to the left of the centerline. It is about five inches long, about three to four inches wide and about three inches thick. The heart is subdivided into four sections: the top two sections are called the *right* and *left atriums*; the two lower sections are called the *right* and *left ventricles*.

Blood from all over the body (except the lungs) returns to the right atrium through the veins. The three main veins that transport the blood back to the right atrium are the *superior vena*, returning blood from the top part of the body; the *inferior vena cava*, returning blood from the bottom part of the body; and the *coronary sinus*, returning blood from the walls of the heart. Let's follow the path of the blood as it travels through the heart. From the right atrium the blood is pushed into the right ventricle. The right ventricle shoots the blood into the *pulmonary trunk*, which transfers the blood into the lungs via two arteries. Once in the lungs, carbon dioxide is left behind for exhalation and oxygen is picked up for oxidation. The pulmonary veins carry the blood back to the left atrium. It is then transferred to the left ventricle and returned to the rest of the body via the *aorta artery*. Valves in each chamber of the heart prevent the blood from going back into each chamber. The heart controls the circulating blood by this process.

THE DIAPHRAGM

The diaphragm is the flexible, dome-shaped muscle that separates the chest cavity above from the abdominal cavity below. It forms the bottom of the thoracic cavity and rests on the liver, stomach, spleen and left kidney.

Assimilation, elimination, respiration, movement, digestion and heartbeat are all dependent on the proper functioning of the diaphragm. It goes virtually unnoticed, yet does some of the body's most important work. As the diaphragm expands and contracts, it stabilizes our bodily functions. With every inhalation, the diaphragm contracts and descends into the abdominal cavity. As it descends, all the internal organs—liver, kidneys, large intestine, small intestine, stomach, pancreas, spleen and gall bladder—are stimulated, massaged and supplied with fresh blood. When the diaphragm descends it also allows the lungs to fill with air as they expand outward and down into the thoracic cavity. With every exhalation, the diaphragm relaxes and ascends into the chest cavity. As it ascends, air is forced out of the lungs. Without the pumping action of the diaphragm, breathing would cease, resulting in death.

The *aorta artery* (the main artery that carries oxygenated blood from the heart to all parts of the body), the *thoracic duct* (which receives lymph from the head, neck, upper left chest and the entire body below the ribs) and the *esophagus* (an empty muscular tube that joins the mouth and nasal passages with the stomach) all pass through the diaphragm. The *vagus nerve*, which authorizes parasympathetic stimulation of the heart, lungs, abdominal organs and esophagus, also passes through the diaphragm. When you run, walk or bend, the *psoas* and *quadratus lumborum* muscles are in use. They attach to the spine, hip and femur, in between the diaphragm and spinal column.

As you can see, the diaphragm assists your entire body to function normally. When the diaphragm becomes restricted, the body begins to malfunction by negatively altering your eliminative, digestive, circulatory, sexual and respiratory systems. Lifestyle is an important factor in determining the quality of your diaphragmic function. If you're under a lot of stress at work, take your job home with you every night, work ten hours a day six or seven days a week, are always too busy to enjoy yourself and seem to be always up too high or down too low, you're subjecting yourself to a very unnatural existence. Your body, including your diaphragm, will be storing the negative effects of your lifestyle. Usually, the beating of the heart is synchronized to the movement of the diaphragm; however, when illness is present this pattern is altered, resulting in poor functioning. If no correction is made and the diaphragm continues to hold this tension, the entire body will suffer due to improper breathing. The *Cleansing Breath* is simple to do and will help restore proper breathing. You need to breathe smoothly so the body can relax—when breathing is irregular, tension can cause more serious illness.

THE CLEANSING BREATH

Sit comfortably in a chair or cross-legged on the floor. Close your eyes and relax. Notice the pattern of your breath as you breathe through your nose. Most people only use the upper third of their chest while breathing. This is shallow breathing and does not allow the lungs to reach their full capacity, resulting in poor elimination of carbon dioxide with every exhalation and an insufficient supply of oxygen and *prana*, or lifeforce, as you inhale. Prolonged breathing in this manner keeps the body full of tension and prevents the brain from receiving its needed supply of oxygen. The brain comprises only about seven percent of the body mass but it uses 25 percent of all the oxygen consumed, so it's vital that we receive enough oxygen for all our needs.

Ever notice children as they breathe? They maximize their lung capacity by naturally breathing deeply and completely. This is your goal. Breathing should always occur through the nose. The nose has two functions: the *vestibule* (outer cavity of the nose) contains coarse hairs that act as a filter and prevent dust particles from entering the body as you breathe. The rest of the nose is lined with mucous membranes that warm the incoming air and also trap dust particles. Thus, incoming air channeled through the nose is purified and warmed, making it easier on the lungs. As you begin to inhale through your nose, let your abdomen fill up with air. If this is difficult to do, place your hand on your abdomen as you inhale and breathe into your hand. Slowly expand the inhalation up to your midchest, then your upper chest. You'll immediately notice that your lung capacity has increased tremendously!

Now as you exhale, slowly draw your abdomen in, expelling all the carbon dioxide. Repeat this cleansing breath for three to five minutes twice a day—once in the morning and again at night. Eventually work up to about 15 minutes each session. Besides experiencing increased lung capacity, you will notice how your mind will slow down and relax. For many people, the clear thinking that results is the greatest gift. Understanding the relationship between body, mind and soul is the key to living a healthy, peaceful, long life. Too often we only relate to our existence through the physical world, without ever honoring our true spiritual center, the true source of all our experiences. Ideally the soul controls the mind and the mind controls the body. The body does nothing but follow orders and is used by the mind to fulfill the soul's wishes. When the mind creates energy blocks in the body and imbalances occur, the body in turn disturbs the function of the mind with pain. Pain is a signal that something isn't functioning properly, and if nothing is done to correct the imbalance, disease can set in. The disease process can be reversed only when we decide to do it ourselves. And for many people, quieting the mind so they can listen to the soul is the first step.

TECHNIQUE TO BALANCE THE DIAPHRAGM

This treatment makes contact with each electrical pole of the diaphragm as it is represented in the body, including reflexes to the feet, hands, ears and head. In this way we hope to stimulate and balance all aspects of the diaphragm, so it can return to normal function.

In the torso the shoulders are the positive pole, the diaphragm the neutral pole and the hips the negative pole. When we view the diaphragm as the negative pole, the shoulders become the neutral pole and the head the positive pole. When the diaphragm is the positive pole, the hips are the neutral pole and the knees the negative pole. We begin with some floor exercises designed to loosen the corresponding diaphragmic electrical poles. First, we squat, which reunites us with the energy fields that were important to us as we developed in the womb. Gently bouncing in the squating position helps to open the hips (see exercise chapter).

1. Skull Traction

Gently lift the head with your left hand and place your right hand beneath the head. Then place your left hand over the forehead, above the eyebrows. Hold for one to three minutes. This will balance the brain and nervous system, inducing deep relaxation.

2. Occipital Ridge to Top of Head

Locate any tension along the occipital ridge at the base of the skull with a gentle massage of the area. Place your fire finger on any tender spot and hold gently. With the ether finger of your other hand, move to the top of the head and make contact on the opposite side from your contact on the occipital ridge. Hold for one or two minutes. This will release the tension at the occipital ridge and relax all the muscles that connect

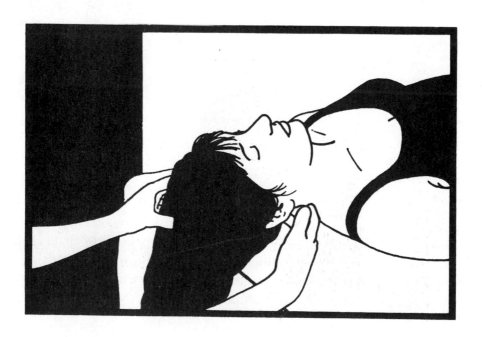

there. If there are other sore spots along the ridge on that side, repeat until they all melt away.

3. Cerebrospinal Pump

Gently lift the head up so that you can place both hands under it with thumbs on the inside of the ears and fingers under the skull. Gently lift the head so that the chin touches the chest. This will lengthen the muscles along the back of the neck and shorten the muscles in the front of the neck. Now reverse the stretch so that the chin is pointing straight up and the top of the head is on the table. Repeat five times. This pumping action activates the cerebrospinal fluid from the brain and sends it down the spinal column. Cerebrospinal fluid contains proteins, glucose, urea, salts and some white blood cells. It functions as a shock absorber for the nervous system by filling in the space around the brain and spinal column. There are approximately four ounces of this fluid in the system at any given time, and as it moves down the spine, it clears out blocks.

4. Shoulder Shake

Place both hands, palms open, on the *trapezius muscles* on top of the shoulders. Alternately move each hand toward the feet by pushing on the shoulder. As you gently shake your client, their head should move slightly from

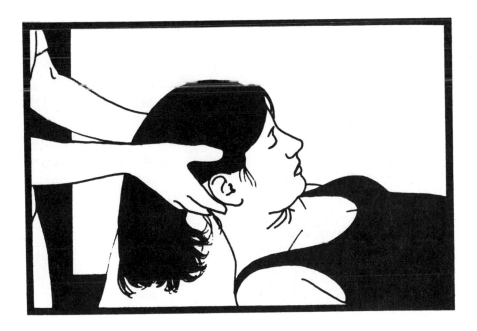

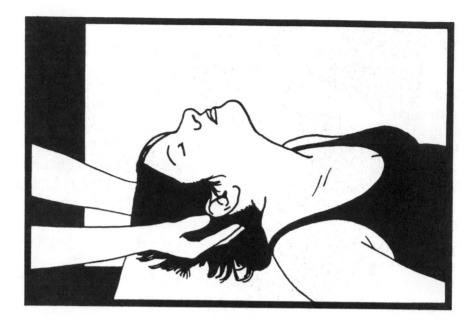

side to side. This will show you that the manipulation is working properly. Shake for about one minute, then pause. Repeat three times. This manipulation begins to break up the tension in the shoulders, which is one of the energy fields of the diaphragm. Your client will immediately notice that they are holding unnecessary tension in their shoulders and let it go.

5. Clavicle Rock

Move to the right side of the table. Place the ether and air fingers of your upper hand on either side of the mid-clavicle, or collar bone. Place the thumb of your lower hand below the *sternum* (breast bone) as the rest of the fingers rest on the lower rib cage. Hold the clavicle contact steady as you move your lower hand down the diaphragm (under the rib cage) on the left side to the end of the rib cage, using a rocking motion. Come back to the sternum contact and repeat five times. This will relieve tension and gas that has accumulated along that side. After you break contact, go to the other side of the table and repeat the same move. When you break contact, let your hands come straight up off the torso in a slow, easy manner. You should always leave the client's energy field gently, as this helps the relaxation process.

6. Foot Session

Measure your client's legs and work on the foot of the longest leg first. The short leg indicates an energy block and tightness. When you work

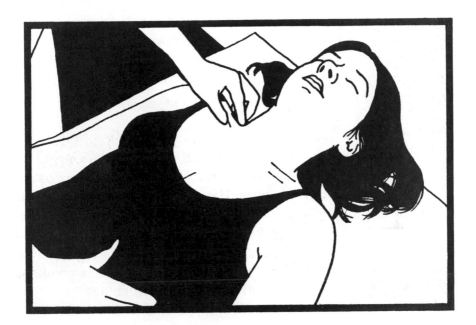

on a foot that is free of energy blocks, the other foot responds sympathet-ically and begins to clear out. If both feet are the same length, work on the right foot first.

A. *Lean and Pull.* Place your outside hand underneath the foot and your inside hand on the ball of the foot. Push the foot back with your inside hand, then place your inside hand on the top of the foot, pulling back the opposite way. Repeat four times. Note that a sore spot on the top of the ankle can represent tension in the diaphragm.

B. *Ankle Rotation.* With your inside hand hold your client's big toe and with your outside hand hold the back of the ankle. Rotate the ankle by rotating the big toe to the left, then to the right—ten times each way. This will help relax all the currents in the foot.

C. *Brachial Plexus Reflex.* With your thumbs, work the area around the ball of the big toe. It reflexes to the *brachial plexus* (the area between the shoulder blades). Continue to work around the entire ball of the foot, us-ing your thumbs. This area reflexes to the heart and lungs. Sometimes there is a great deal of tenderness at these points, and it usually feels very good to have them worked out.

D. *Tendon Reflex.* The tendons in between the first and second *metatar-sals* of the feet reflex to the diaphragm and brachial plexus. Usually this part of the body is very tender to the touch, so be gentle as you begin to place your thumb there and slide it up and down the tendon. Stay in touch with your client and have them breathe through any sore or tender spot. Breathing reunites the body to the soul. It bridges the physical world to the spiritual world and has a transforming effect on everyone.

E. *Foot Element Balancing.* (See foot treatment, pages 48–53.)

7. Diaphragm-to-Foot Contact

Place your thumb on top of the ankle where the *talus* (ankle bone) meets the *tibia* and *fibula* (the two long bones of the lower leg) and let your fingers make contact around the ankle bone. Have your upper hand make contact with the diaphragm, just below the rib cage on the same side. Alternately stimulate each contact for about 30 seconds each. Repeat three or four times and then perform the same manipulation on the other side. The thumb contact on top of the ankle is a diaphragm reflex point and is usually sore in people with breathing or chest difficulties.

8. Diaphragm Sweep

Start on the right side of the table. Place your upper hand on the diaphragm by the liver and your lower hand on the hip. Rock both contacts gently for one minute. Now move your lower hand to the knee on the same side and rock both contacts for one minute. Go to the other side and repeat the same moves.

9. Diaphragm-to-Ear Contact

Stand on the right side of your client and place your right hand on the right side of the diaphragm by the liver. Place your left hand on the shoulder and gently rock both contacts for one minute. Pause for about half a minute, then repeat three times. Now break contact with your left hand and move it up to the ear contact on the diaphragm line, which is located about a half inch below the top of the ear. Hold for one minute. The ear contact may be a little tender. Repeat both contacts on the other side.

10. Cardiac Stability Hold

Stand on the right side of the table. Place your right hand over the midsternum with fingers pointing toward the head. Place your left earth finger over the ear and your thumb on the third eye. Let the rest of the fingers fall into place between the two. Hold for two to three minutes. This will balance the heartbeat to the rhythm of the lungs, restoring proper function.

11. Scapula Release

Stand behind your client and have them roll to either side. Bring their arm behind their back, exposing the *scapula,* or shoulder blade. Place one hand under the scapula and the other hand on the front of the shoulder. Have your client take a deep breath, and on the exhalation, lift with both hands. Repeat three times. This will stretch the immobile muscles in the brachial plexus and bring wonderful relief. Then have your client roll to the other side and repeat the manipulation.

12. Sacrum-to-Neck Contact

Move to the right side of the table. Place your right hand over the sacrum, or pelvis, and your left hand behind the neck. Hold for three minutes. This will end the treatment on a balanced note.

Many things can manifest during this treatment. It is a very active one and usually stirs up old emotions or recall of events that have been stored deeply inside. Be prepared for intense releases manifesting as crying, cursing, etc. Lung capacity should be increased at least 25 percent and normal breathing restored. I have used this treatment many times with wonderful results.

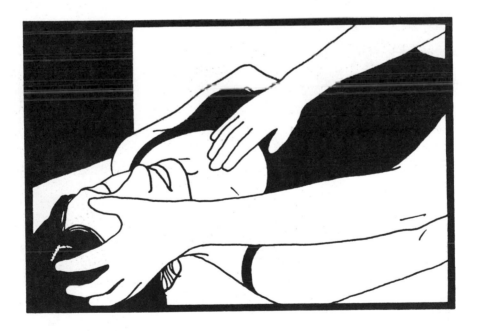

THE FIRE ELEMENT

The Fire Element represents the warmth and heat in the body, which is derived from the digestion of foods and liquids. The body needs constant stimulation to rid itself of accumulated wastes, and the Fire Element provides the necessary strength to accomplish this. This is best demonstrated by the action of certain foods and spices like cayenne pepper, garlic or ginger. These foods stimulate the blood tremendously, increase heat and warmth in the body and improve circulation. They give the entire system a boost which enables it to do its work more effectively.

The three poles of the Fire Element in the body are: Aries, the eyes, the Ram's charging energy, the positive pole; Leo the Lion, the solar plexus, the rebuilder of strength, the neutral pole; and Sagittarius the Archer, the power of the thighs, the negative pole. When the Fire Element combines with the other elements, certain qualities are manifested. Hunger is the dominating characteristic of the Fire Element. When the Fire Element combines with the Ether Element, sleep is manifested. When the Fire Element combines with the Air Element, thirst is created. When the Fire Element combines with the Water Element, luster is formed. When the Fire Element combines with the Earth Element, laziness is created.

The best ways to activate the Fire Element in the body are touch, food and exercise. When we touch someone in a "fiery" way, we touch them actively. There are many foods that can be classified as fiery, such as cayenne pepper, garlic, onions, ginger, and all the grains—rice, millet, oats and kasha. The old expression, "He's feeling his oats," meaning being full of energy, describes the Fire Element. These foods are a tonic for the circulatory system; they stimulate the blood and create more warmth and action. The exercises called "Woodchopper" and "Ha-Frog" (see pages 137–138) also get the blood moving. It is good to get your clients involved in these exercises so they can help themselves.

You wouldn't want to do a Fire session on someone who has cancer, boils, fever, rashes of any kind or any internal inflammation. You would want to do a Fire session on someone who is low in energy, always tired, emotional, feeling depressed or has any digestive disorder. Also, the Fire session helps the eliminative process, especially constipation or diarrhea.

The digestive system requires many organs to do its work, and it is important to know the path the food takes as it travels through the digestive tract.

WHAT HAPPENS TO FOOD IN THE BODY

Food goes through four major chemical changes during digestion. The first step is in the mouth, where saliva begins to break down starches in an alkaline, non-acid medium. In the stomach, proteins are digested by hydrochloric acid and an enzyme called *pepsin*. The breaking down of proteins is slow and usually takes at least two hours. The *chyme* (semifluid mixture of partly digested food) then journeys to the first part of the small intestine, called the *duodenum*. Enzymes from the *pancreas* enter the duodenum and complete the job the mouth began by breaking down the remaining starches. *Bile* (an enzyme secreted by the liver and stored in the gall bladder) is also secreted into the duodenum from the *gall bladder*, and begins to break down fat. The pancreas also secretes enzymes that complete the breakdown of fats, proteins and carbohydrates. The small intestine has an alkaline medium: most of the digestive process is completed there. As the chyme continues on through the small intestinal tract, nutrients are absorbed through the walls of the *villi* into the *portal vein*, which goes directly to the *liver*. The liver is the main chemical plant of the body and filters out all the toxins. It also stores sugar to be used by the body at a future time. The blood, rich in nutrients, continues on to the heart and lungs. The semisolid unused fiber that remains is passed on through to the large intestine via the *ileocecal valve*. About 90 percent of the water is absorbed in the large intestine. Bacterial growth changes the remaining semisolid mass into *feces* so it can be eliminated through the *anus*. These helpful bacteria need an acid environment to grow in and the large intestine provides that medium.

TECHNIQUE TO BALANCE THE FIRE ELEMENT

Throughout the Fire treatment, the hand on the umbilical center should provide a stimulating contact. As you make contacts along the body, try to have your thumbs facing each other, creating a current that will spread the energy from the navel center all over the body and greatly uplift the energy level of your client.

1. Fire Center Stimulation

Have your client lie on their back. Move to their right side and find the umbilicus (navel); move down about an inch, and over about an inch to the right. With your thumb, in an up and down motion, stimulate the area for about one minute, then hold gently for about one minute. Repeat this process three times. While you are doing this, the thumb of your other hand should contact the third eye lightly.

2. Fire Above

Slowly break the contact on the third eye; with that same hand move to the liver contact below the rib cage on the right side. With your right hand, continue stimulating the umbilical area. Then move your left hand to the contacts along the clavicle: mid-jaw, sinus point below the eye, orbital ridge; then back down along the other side and finish at the spleen contact below the rib cage on the left side. Hold each contact for at least one minute.

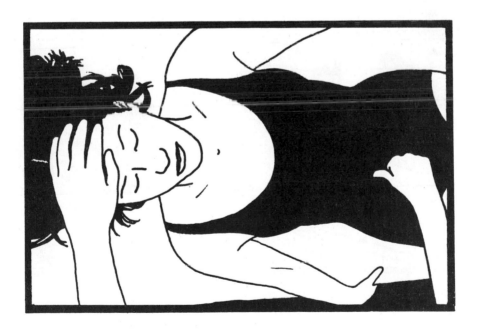

3. Fire Below

Switch hands and move down so that your left hand is now making contact at the umbilical center. With your right hand, contact the mid-thigh point on each thigh, the knee points right above each knee and then the foot points on the mid-foot (air finger on top and ether finger on the bottom of the foot).

4. Leo-Sagittarius Rock

Place one hand on the torso side of your client's hip and the other hand on the knee. Rock both contacts, then slowly move the hand on the knee up and down the thigh. Repeat on the other side (see illustration below). Leo represents the solar plexus and Sagittarius the thighs.

5. Fire Finger to Fire Toe

Hold the fire finger of one hand and the fire toe of the corresponding foot for two minutes. Repeat on the other side. Brush off.

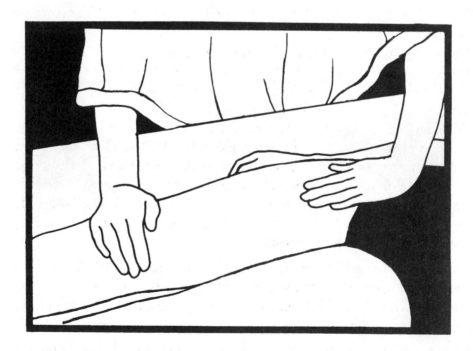

THE WATER ELEMENT

The planet Earth and the human body consist of about 75—80 percent water. We relate to our physical body so completely we forget that our true essence is vibrational and that it holds us together. The Water Element flows through us in the form of saliva, urine, blood, semen, mucus, sweat, cerebrospinal fluid and phlegm. Our fluids have a natural downward flow to our feet. The Water Element is the body's foundation: our equilibrium and balance are maintained by a harmonious water level.

The Water Element rules our creativity and sexuality. The three poles of the Water Element in the body are: Cancer, the breasts and lymph glands, the positive pole; Scorpio, the genitals, the neutral pole; and Pisces, the feet, the negative pole. The production of semen is the dominant characteristic of the Water Element. When the Water Element combines with the Ether Element, saliva is formed. When the Water Element combines with the Air Element, sweat is formed. When the Water Element combines with the Fire Element, urine is formed. When the Water Element combines with the Earth Element, blood is formed. The Water Element is represented by movement. When we touch someone in a deep way, it keeps the energy moving.

Some foods that are classified as "watery" are: leafy vegetables, melons, cucumbers, squash, honey, watery fruits and milk. Salty foods are considered watery. The "Cliffhanger" exercise (see page 138) moves a lot of energy very quickly.

I don't believe in deep work, and as a rule, I never work deeply on anyone. Deep work can activate a quick detoxification throughout the entire body, but many unforeseen emotional reactions can occur for up to 24 hours afterwards, leaving your client with the burden of dealing with them without necessarily being ready or willing to do so. Besides, most people don't want to be hurt. Remember, the most important aspect of Polarity Therapy is to use the love energy. Force is the opposite of love; let force remain dormant!

TECHNIQUE TO BALANCE THE WATER ELEMENT

By working on the feet, the long currents of the body are returned to their proper patterns. Before you start, gently place both hands on your client's feet. Bring the feet together, lift them about a foot in the air and rotate them three times. Place the ankles together and measure them. The short side indicates a block, so you should begin on the longer leg. The feet do not distinguish between right and left, so both of them are affected at the same time. By working on the unblocked side first, you send some energy to the blocked side, so that it will be easier to work on. If the ankles measure the same, start on the right side, the more active, yang side.

1. Lean and Pull

Place your outside hand underneath the foot and your inside hand on the ball of the foot. Push the foot back with your inside hand, then place your inside hand on the top of the foot, pulling back the opposite way. Repeat

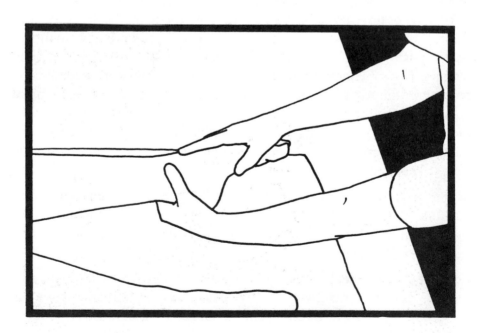

four times. A sore spot on the top of the ankle can represent tension in the diaphragm.

2. Ankle Rotation

With your inside hand hold your client's big toe and with your outside hand hold the back of the ankle. Rotate the ankle by rotating the big toe to the left, then to the right—ten times each way. This will help relax all the currents in the foot.

3. Inside Ankle Point

With your outside hand, bring your client's foot outside with the toes toward the table, giving access to the inside ankle. With your thumb, stimulate the area below the ankle bone for about 30 seconds, then hold gently. Repeat three times. This contact stimulates the single organs of the reproductive system: a man's penis and a woman's womb.

4. Outside Ankle Point

Bend the foot toward the inside of your client's body, revealing the outside of the ankle. Stimulate the point just under the ankle bone, then hold gently. Repeat three times.

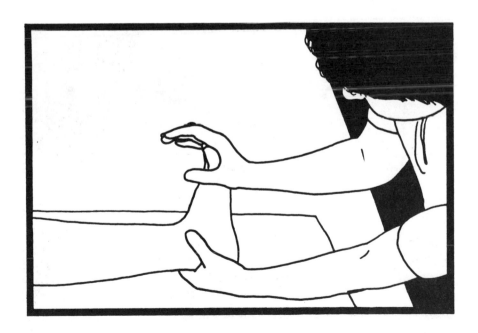

5. Knuckle Rub

This contact stimulates the double organs of the reproductive system: testes in men and ovaries in women. Make a fist with one hand; with your knuckles rub the sole of your client's foot up and down. Your other hand is placed on top of the foot for support. Repeat ten times. This will also stimulate most of the major organs that have reflexes on the soles of the feet (refer to foot chart, page 53).

6. Flexed Big Tendon

Place your thumb on the ball of your client's foot at the base of the big toe. Place your other hand on top of the foot for support. Flex down on the toes and press in on the tendon, holding a few seconds, then release. Repeat this contact three times as you move down along the tendon, every half inch to the bottom of the foot. This works on the Ether Element as well as the spine.

7. Toe Pulls

Place your thumbs on top of your client's ankle and slowly move down toward the toes, in between each tendon. Hold the toe at its base with your ether finger on top and your air finger on the bottom; slowly wiggle

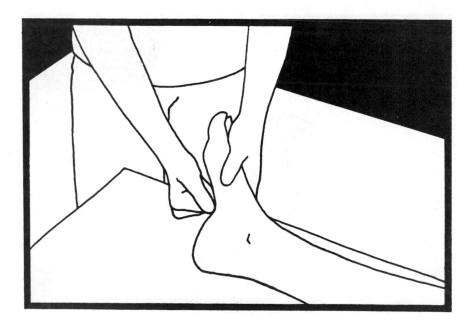

and pull the toe toward you at the same time. Often the toe will pop; if it doesn't, just go on to the next one. This gets the blocked energy moving and stimulates all five elements in the body.

8. Tootsie Rolls

Place both hands around each of your client's toes and slide back and forth, rolling the toe from side to side, about 30 seconds for each toe.

9. Spine Flex

With the ether and air fingers of your outside hand, contact the first joint of the big toe; with the thumb of your other hand, slowly move along the arch of the foot, from the base of the big toe to the heel. Repeat three times. The arch of the foot represents the spine; any sore spot correlates to soreness along the spine.

10. Toe Brushing

Hold your client's foot firmly with one hand while the palm of your other hand skims along the very top of the toes. Repeat ten times. This stimulates the energy at the very end of its current and greatly promotes its return upward.

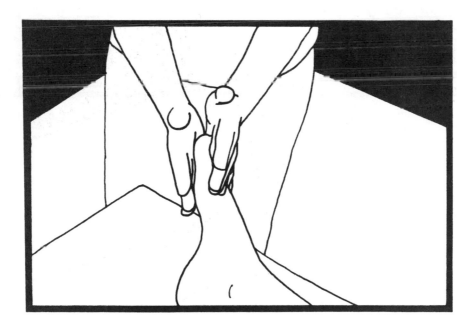

11. Foot Element Balancing

Place your thumb on the inside ankle point, with your fist closed. With the air finger of your other hand, gently contact the top of each toe for about one minute. Quite often during this sequence, your client will have tremendous releases; all the other foot moves you've done are being assimilated at this time.

When you've finished, place both hands on your client's calf and slowly move down and off the foot. This will remove any excess energy.

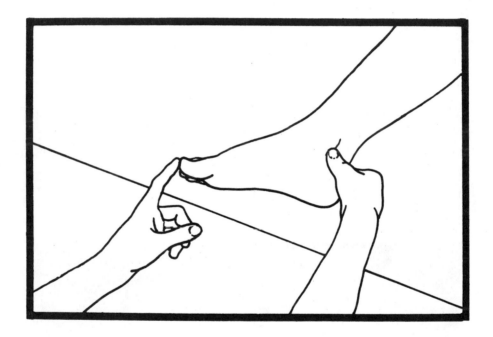

REFLEXOLOGY and ACU-POINTS
RIGHT FOOT

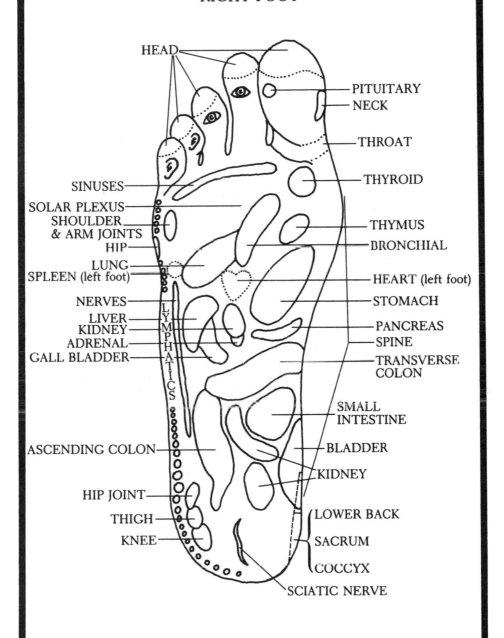

HEAD

PITUITARY

NECK

THROAT

THYROID

SINUSES

SOLAR PLEXUS

SHOULDER
& ARM JOINTS

HIP

LUNG

SPLEEN (left foot)

THYMUS

BRONCHIAL

HEART (left foot)

NERVES

LIVER

KIDNEY

ADRENAL

GALL BLADDER

STOMACH

PANCREAS

SPINE

TRANSVERSE
COLON

LYMPHATICS

SMALL
INTESTINE

ASCENDING COLON

BLADDER

KIDNEY

HIP JOINT

THIGH

KNEE

LOWER BACK

SACRUM

COCCYX

SCIATIC NERVE

THE EARTH ELEMENT

The Earth Element is what gives structure and support to your body. Hair, skin, bones, flesh, muscles and nails manifest through the Earth Element. Foods containing carbon, such as honey, sugar, fats, dairy products, animal products, starches and carbohydrates are classified with the Earth Element because they are stored as fat. All foods that grow below the ground, like tubers, are considered of the Earth family because they grow in the earth.

The main manifestation of the Earth Element in our bodies is the *skeletal system*, which supports us against gravity and holds our muscles and organs together. The formation of bones is the main function of the Earth Element in the body. Hair is formed when the Ether Element joins with the Earth Element. Skin is formed when the Air Element joins with the Earth Element. Blood vessels are formed when the Fire Element joins with the Earth Element. Flesh is formed when the Water Element joins with the Earth Element.

The three poles of the Earth Element are: Taurus the Bull, located in the neck area, the positive pole; Virgo the Virgin, the bowels, the neutral pole; and Capricorn the Goat, the knees, the negative pole.

Earth foods are easy to assimilate but difficult to eliminate. We crave Earth foods because our bodies want to store these essential elements to be used as fuel when needed. This excess buildup of food is stored as fat. The function of the colon determines our eliminative capability, and is ruled by the Earth Element. Fear, calmness, contraction, laziness, greed, possessiveness, envy, stability and forgiveness are all qualities of the Earth Element.

THE LARGE INTESTINE

The large intestine is the principal organ of digestion. It is about five feet in length and two and one-half inches in diameter. It is a continuation of the small intestine, beginning at the *ileum* and extending to the anus. The four major sections of the large intestine are the *cecum, colon, rectum*, and *anal canal*. The ileum meets the large intestine at the *ileocecal valve*, which allows the chyme from the small intestine to move into the large intestine. The cecum is about three inches long and hangs below the ileocecal valve. The *appendix* attaches to the downward end of the cecum, while the colon joins the other end. The colon is like a long hose divided into four major parts: the *ascending colon, transverse colon, descending colon* and *sigmoid colon*. It makes a sharp left turn across the abdomen to the lower end of the *spleen*; this is called the transverse colon. Then it makes a sharp right turn down to the *iliac crest* (the top of the hipbone); this is the descending colon. The sigmoid colon begins at the iliac crest and moves toward the middle of the body, completing its journey at the rectum. The opening at the end of the rectum is the anus.

Peristalsis, a wavelike action within a muscular tube, is the movement within the large intestine that pushes the food along its tract. *Absorption*, the passing of nutrients from chyme into the blood, usually takes from three to eight hours. What remains is called *feces* and is pushed along until it is eliminated through the anus. The absorption of water occurs at the cecum and ascending colon and assists in maintaining a balanced water level. To help the chyme decompose, an alkaline solution is secreted that assists the bacteria in their fermentation process, with gas as a by-product.

PROBLEMS IN THE LARGE INTESTINE

The large intestine is the sewer system of the body and its proper function is essential for good health. Any difficulty there will slow elimination, causing a host of problems, like a sewer pipe that backs up or overflows. Constipation arises when too much water is absorbed from the feces, resulting in difficult and infrequent elimination. Diarrhea develops when not enough water is absorbed from the feces, resulting in loose, frequent bowel movements. Fear and anxiety can disrupt the interaction of the bacteria with the chyme in the large intestine, resulting in excess gas that can travel throughout the system, causing pain. Dr. Stone discusses this problem and says that this gas can also lodge itself in bones, the brain, the spinal column, muscles and the internal organs. The following is a list of symptoms that can be caused by excess gas in the system:

1. Chronic migraine headaches
2. Shooting pains throughout the body
3. Cramps in the calves
4. Pain in the bowels
5. Pain in the bones
6. Numbness in the arms after a heavy meal
8. Cramps
9. Hiccoughs: can be gas pressure on the diaphragm.

A diet that is high in processed food, pollutants from our environment, a lifestyle that constantly swings from high to low and back again, over-eating, drinking after meals, eating the wrong food combinations and using drugs can all have negative effects on absorption and elimination, creating many physical problems.

COLONIC THERAPY

To counteract any build-up of gas and to tonify the colon, you want to encourage the downward drainage and expulsion impulse. Colonic or enema therapy is recommended to empty out the bowels. The only restriction is during pregnancy, as any sudden elimination could hurt the fetus. During a colonic, a rubber hose is inserted into the anus. Pressurized warm water is released into the bowels and travels into the colon. When the pressure reaches a certain point, it is released, and fecal matter accompanies the water as it is expelled. This process continues for one hour and is very effective in cleansing the entire colon. Usually a series of colonics is recommended because old fecal matter can stick to the walls of the colon and needs to be loosened before it can be expelled. Colonics should only be administered by trained therapists. If you decide on colonic therapy, seek out a professional who has a good reputation. It is a delicate therapy, but you can achieve excellent results with a trained practitioner whom you trust.

Enema therapy can be self-administered with the use of an enema bag that you can purchase at any pharmacy. Fill a two-quart bag with warm water and hang it no higher than two feet above you. If the bag is higher than two feet, there can be too much pressure created by gravity and this can cause unnecessary pain. Lubricate the end of the plastic hose and gently insert it into the anus. Release the flow of water from the valve and wait until you feel pressure build up, then close the valve. You should be in the bathroom, so that the water can be expelled immediately. The longer you can hold the water in, the more powerful the effect. While administering an enema, you should be on your knees with your head leaning forward. By gently rolling from side to side while the enema is being administered, you can cause the water to come up higher into the transverse colon. Repeat this process until there is no more fecal matter expelled. This is usually accomplished after three bags of water. Remember to sterilize your equipment in alcohol after each use. Colonics and enemas are more powerful when you fast, as they speed up the elimination of toxins. They should not be administered after a meal. As the colon is cleansed, peristaltic activity will return to normal, fecal matter that has lodged against the colon's lining will be discharged, resulting in a feeling of lightness, and chyme will pass through easier.

HEALING CRISES

From quickly removing the many energy blocks and toxins stored in the colon, a healing crisis may develop. During a healing crisis the individual may suddenly become ill. A slight fever, cramps, chills, tiredness, a headache, the blahs, can all be symptoms of a healing crisis. But these will usually pass in a short time and the individual will feel better.

A healing crisis can also develop from receiving hands-on bodywork. The releasing of energy blocks manifests differently in each individual. Crying, screaming, yelling, grunting and cursing are some of the ways people expel energy blocks. Getting in touch with past traumas, recalling negative experiences with former loved ones, past-life regression, letting go of old emotions and dealing with a broken heart are some of the experiences I have helped people get through during a treatment. The bodywork aspect of Polarity Therapy is a very powerful experience: you can watch people cut through many layers of hang-ups in a relatively short time.

Make yourself available to your clients, especially when you suggest a quick detoxification. Don't recommend a colonic and then be too busy to be there if they need you. This can leave them in a difficult situation, so if you encourage people to detoxify, make sure you are available to help them through any healing crises.

DIETARY THERAPY

If colonic therapy seems too radical for your client, a dietary change is a gentler approach that can bring about wonderful results. To stop diarrhea, add a little cinnamon to a crushed apple. Dehydration can result from excessive diarrhea (especially in little children), so it's important to consume lots of liquids and watch the fluid level in the body. Constipation can be cured by consuming prune and fig juice, soaked dried fruits, bran, brown rice and leafy vegetables and by squatting. If constipation is a constant problem, a dietary change is recommended. Stop eating red meat, as it is very difficult to digest and can stay in the digestive system for up to two weeks as it ferments. If you feel you are stuck in your life situation, your job or a relationship, constipation can result. It can also be caused by continuous overeating. What comes to mind is a backed-up sewer drain: it can't handle the amount of sewage going through it, so it slows down. The same thing happens in the body when you consume large amounts of food that are hard to digest. At this point you must determine what your relationship with food really is and see how food may represent many things to you besides fuel for your body. Observing when and why you eat is the first step toward slowing down the overeating habit. *Eat only when you are hungry*. If you can master this concept, your overeating will cease and your body will function efficiently again. Don't eat because you are sad, bored, feel unloved, insecure, depressed, overworked or anxious. Those are the wrong reasons to put food into your system, and consuming food in this manner will create many energy blocks in your body.

TECHNIQUE TO BALANCE THE LARGE INTESTINE

This treatment uses both a chair and table and is divided into two parts. Start by having your client sit down straddling a chair.

1. Skull Traction

Stand behind your client to the left. Gently place your left hand horizontally with your fingers on their forehead above the eyebrows and your right hand on the back of their neck. Hold for three minutes. This hold will balance the nervous system, release tension in the head and bring a feeling of lightness and relaxation.

2. Waist Rock

Stand behind your client and gently place both hands on the side of their hips with your thumbs touching the lower lumbar vertebra and your fingers above the groin over the ascending and descending colon (as if encircling the hips). Rock gently. This will release accumulated gas in the colon and should be continued for three to five minutes.

3. Shoulder Rock

Stand behind your client and place both hands over their shoulders with your fingers stimulating the area in front of the collar bone and your thumbs along the trapezius muscles. Rock gently for one minute, pause, and repeat three times.

4. Spinal Flex

Stand behind your client and place both thumbs on the muscles along either side of the spinal column, but not directly on the spine. Now slowly move down the spine, stimulating each vertebra, one by one. Start at the neck and finish at the sacrum (hips). Repeat three times.

5. Head Rock

From behind, place both hands on either side of your client's skull. Lightly rock the head from hand to hand as you move over the skull. Work out any sore spots you find. This will release any gas pressure that may have accumulated in the skull.

6. Head Cradle

Have your client lie down on the table on their back. Choose any head cradle you know and hold for one to three minutes. This will balance the nervous system and bring deep relaxation quickly.

7. Tibia Contact

Stand on the right side of your client by their leg. Locate the *tibia* (shin bone) and place your ether and air fingers on either side of it. Start where the tibia joins the ankle bone and slowly move up toward the knee as you firmly stimulate each side of the tibia, inch by inch. Stay in touch with your client and locate any tender or sore spots. Hold firmly on any tender spot, then continue upward. This contact reflexes the ascending colon until about four inches from the knee. At this point you are on the transverse colon for the right side of the body. After you locate tender spots along the tibia, make a similar contact between the *ulna* and *radius* of the arm (forearm bones). These are the colon reflexes of the arm and correspond directly to the reflexes of the legs. Now your lower hand has a contact on the tibia of the leg, while your upper hand makes contact between the ulna and radius of the arm. For best results wiggle each contact simultaneously. You will notice that a tender spot on the leg is usually matched by one on the arm. If the pain is greater on the leg contact it means that the imbalance in the large intestine is chronic and has been

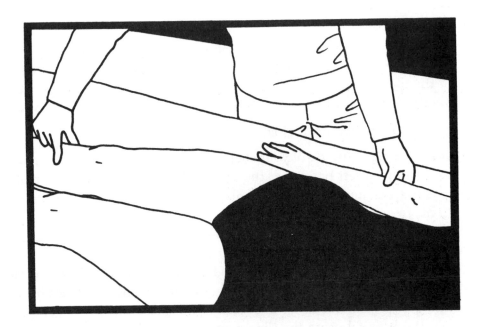

there for a long time. If the pain is greater on the arm contact, it means that the condition is acute or a recent occurrence.

8. Tibia-to-Torso Contact

Stand on the right side of the table and locate tender spots along the tibia as you did in move #7. After they are located, place your upper hand directly on the colon at that point. The torso contact should be tender. Alternately stimulate each contact with a wiggle. Repeat three times.

9. Arm-to-Torso Contact

Contact the tender spots along the arm between the ulna and radius. After they are located, place your other hand directly on the colon at its corresponding point. Wiggle each contact. Repeat for all tender spots you find. Repeat manipulations 7, 8 and 9 on the left side of the body for the transverse and descending colon reflexes.

10. Foot Rub

Give a foot rub, emphasizing the colon reflexes, which are located in the center of the sole of the foot. Do both feet.

11. Colon Drain

Stand on the right side of the table. Place both hands on your client's abdomen with fingers spread out and fingertips facing one another. Firmly twist the loose stomach tissue counter-clockwise. This is a digestive and bowel stimulant because it reverses the normal flow. Repeat three times.

12. Abdomen-to-Forehead Hold

Standing to the right side of your client, place your right hand on the abdomen and your left hand over the forehead above the eyebrows. Hold for one to three minutes. This is a balancing hold and will soothe and relax. This treatment is very stimulating and will enhance proper function of the large intestine. Anyone with constipation will usually have a bowel movement within 12 hours after receiving this treatment. It can also help stop diarrhea. Excess gas will be released, bringing relief from pain often caused by this condition. Once a friend of mine, having just given birth, was in a lot of pain because she couldn't pass gas. I worked at her bedside in the hospital using the tibia contact points. Within five minutes she passed the gas and the pain was gone. There are many people who suffer from large intestinal ailments. This treatment can be the beginning of the healing process for them.

SUMMARY OF THE AYURVEDIC THEORY OF THE FIVE ELEMENTS

ELEMENT	Ether	Air	Fire	Water	Earth
SENSE	Hearing	Touching	Seeing	Tasting	Smelling
TASTE		Sour	Bitter	Salty	Sweet
FOODS	Meditation	Acid fruits, nuts, dairy products	Grains, cayenne pepper	Squash, watery fruits	Honey, sweet fruits
BODY PARTS	Spine Nerves Arteries	Shoulders Kidneys Ankles	Head Solar Plexus Thighs	Breasts Generative organs, Feet	Neck Bowels Knees
BODY FUNCTION	Defines body's space	All movement	Digestion & metabolism	Fluids that lubricate	Solid & liquid wastes

THE STOMACH

The stomach is a J-shaped organ located under the diaphragm in the upper part of the left abdominal region. The top of the stomach is connected to the *esophagus* and the bottom to the *duodenum,* or first part of the small intestine. The stomach has great elasticity and can expand to accomodate large amounts of food. After we swallow our food it goes directly into the stomach. With every inhalation, the diaphragm pushes the stomach down and pulls it up with every exhalation, so as we breathe the stomach receives a gentle massage.

The main function of the stomach is to break down proteins, which it does with the help of enzymes and hydrochloric acid. Food is changed into *chyme* (food partly digested by enzymes during digestion) so it can move more easily through the digestive tract. The chyme is helped along its way through the stomach by peristaltic action until it empties into the duodenum. From there it moves through the small intestine and into the large intestine. The stomach secretes mucus that coats its lining and prevents the hydrochloric acid used in digestion from causing a burn. If, however, there isn't enough mucus secreted, the acid can penetrate the stomach wall and cause an ulcer.

Food leaves the stomach from two to four hours after it has been eaten. During a meal with many different kinds of food, it's best to eat the proteins first, followed by the carbohydrates, fats, etc. If you don't follow this order, the other foods will absorb the enzymes meant for the proteins, and when they arrive there will be no enzymes left for their digestion. If you have difficulty digesting your food, try a little acidophilus after you eat. This will help your stomach do its job and also help relieve any upset stomach.

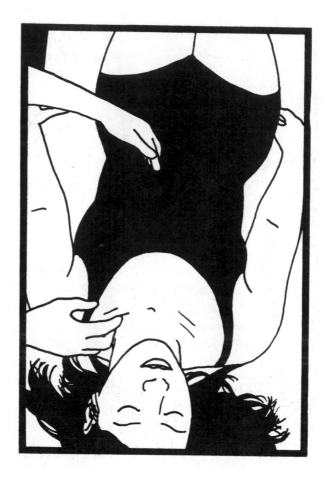

TECHNIQUE TO BALANCE THE STOMACH

Have your client lie on their back. Move to the left side of the table. Place the four fingers of your upper hand under the clavicle. There may be some soreness there, so be gentle. Place the four fingers of your lower hand underneath the floating ribs on the left side. Rock gently for about one minute, then pause for about one minute. Repeat the sequence three times. You might hear some intestinal gurgles from this manipulation. This is a good sign and means the digestive tract is beginning to empty out.

1. Knee-to-Elbow Contact

Place your left hand on the muscles just above the knee. Place your right hand on the muscles just above the elbow. Gently rock each contact for about 30 seconds, then hold for about one minute. Repeat the sequence three times. The knee and elbow on the left side of the body are stomach reflexes, and this manipulation will release any energy block there.

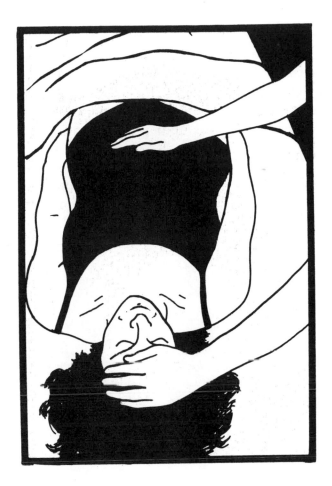

2. Foot-to-Stomach Contact

Move down to the left foot and contact the stomach reflex point on the bottom of the foot. If you suspect that the stomach is out of balance, the foot reflex point may be sore, so be careful not to contact this point too hard or your client may jump off the table. Be gentle but firm in your contact. Many times people respond to sore points with a gasp and a question about the tenderness. If you want to explain it, it's okay to let them know what the point is. Often people will begin to release their energy blocks once they have a confirmation that can be felt. With your right hand, make contact directly over the stomach on the left central lower rib cage. Alternately rock each contact for one minute, then rest for one minute. Repeat this sequence three times. This will help the peristaltic action in the stomach and allow the food to continue its journey.

3. Alternate Shoulder Shake

Move to the right side of the table. Place your right hand over the left hipbone on the ilium. Place your left hand over the right shoulder. Gently rock both hands together for about one minute, then pause for one minute. Repeat this sequence three times. The rocking action will send energy through the stomach and break up any blockage there.

4. Umbilical Center-to-Forehead Contact

Stay on the right side of the table. Place your left hand over the forehead above the eyebrows. Place your right hand over the umbilical center. Hold for three to five minutes. This soft, gentle hold will provide a soothing conclusion to this active treatment.

THE LIVER

The liver is the body's largest glandular organ and lies beneath the diaphragm on the right side of the lower chest. The adult liver weighs approximately four pounds and is separated by the *falciform ligament* into two sections, or *lobes*. Each lobe consists of masses of liver cells joined together into *lobules*. *Sinusoids* are the tiny spaces between the lobules where oxygen, nutrients and poisons are removed from the blood as it passes through.

The liver produces bile, a greenish fluid used by the small intestine in the absorption of fats. The liver stores copper, iron, vitamins A, D, K and E, and *glycogen* (a soluble starch-like substance). It changes glycogen, fat and protein into *glucose* (simple sugar). If the body doesn't need it, it's stored until it does. As the body uses proteins for its energy supply, a toxic waste is produced. The liver converts this waste into urea (a crystallized solid). Urea is eliminated by the kidneys and through the skin. Poisons that can't be eliminated are stored by the liver, which also produces new blood.

In today's world of severe planetary pollution, the earth we grow our food in, the air we breathe and the water we drink have all been contaminated. We are continually being subjected to high levels of poison and have become overly dependent on drugs in an attempt to bring our bodies back into balance. As a result, our livers are overloaded and overworked. Because of this, the liver has a tendency to expand as its capacity to filter toxins decreases. A sluggish liver means sluggish blood, which can lead to many other problems. Overeating puts tremendous pressure on the liver, as it must process more food than it was intended for. The liver grows in size to accomodate the extra food and its function is slowed down. Alcohol, drugs, chemical pesticides, meat, fried foods and vinegar make the liver work harder. They should be avoided in large quantities. By reducing the amount and kinds of foods we consume, we can make sure that the liver, as well as the entire body, won't have to work so hard to digest and assimilate them.

A malfunctioning liver can manifest many symptoms: tiredness, headaches, muscle spasms throughout the body, poor circulation and a tendency to have a long-lasting cold. It can be helped by the following concoction:

THE LIVER FLUSH

1. Two to three tablespoons of cold-pressed olive oil
2. The fresh juice of one lemon
3. Four ozs. of fresh orange juice
4. One or two cloves of fresh garlic
5. A pinch of cayenne pepper

Mix all the ingredients in a blender for one minute. Pour into a glass and drink slowly. If you don't have a blender, place all the ingredients except the garlic into a jar, shake and drink. Eat the garlic separately.

You should consume the Liver Flush within 30 minutes after arising in the morning. Wait another 15 minutes and drink hot lemon tea, consisting of the juice of one freshly squeezed lemon and a cup of hot water. Never use honey or any other sweetner while consuming the Liver Flush. On mornings when you use this drink, don't eat your usual breakfast. By avoiding food the entire digestive tract will get a well-deserved rest and the Liver Flush will be that much more effective. This drink is very filling and you probably won't be hungry afterward. It will also relieve constipation.

Variations: If cold-pressed olive oil is unavailable, use cold-pressed almond oil. Most commercial oils on the market have been heated in processing. Heating changes the molecular structure of the oil, making it difficult for the liver to process. Cold-pressed oils aren't heated and work as an antidote for the liver by drawing out toxins. You may use fresh apple juice instead of orange juice and fresh ginger juice if garlic is not available. Grate the ginger, then squeeze by hand to extract the juice.

The following is a dietary guideline to help keep the liver functioning at its optimum level:

1. Avoid eating fried foods, as they are usually prepared in oil that has been heated to about 400 degrees. The liver has a difficult time trying to break down such fat-soaked food.
2. Avoid consuming large amounts of sugar. The liver converts sugar to glycogen and stores it for further use. Overconsumption of sugar makes

the liver work harder and longer in producing glycogen. When the liver is kept busy processing too much sugar or fried food it can't perform its main function, which is processing all the nutrients it receives from the intestinal tract. Toxins won't be filtered out but will remain in the blood to circulate throughout the body. Some of the unfiltered wastes that remain in the blood can contaminate and directly affect the function of the brain and nervous system, resulting in depression and a feeling of being stuck.

3. Avoid overeating. Too many nutrients flooding the liver tend to weaken it.

4. Avoid eating too many refined foods. Refined foods are absorbed quickly and force the liver to work very hard to process this rapid assimilation.

5. Avoid drinking liquids after a meal. Liquids keep the stomach from properly preparing the chyme. The liver then receives a watered-down version of the food and must work hard to compensate for it.

TECHNIQUE TO BALANCE THE LIVER

This technique will begin to clear out any blockage in the liver that might be causing it to perform sluggishly. You can include these manipulations within the structure of a treatment or use them separately.

1. Floating Rib-to-Clavicle Contact

Stand on the right side of the table with your client on their back. Place all four fingers of your right hand midway under the floating rib on the right side. Place all four fingers of your left hand under the top of the clavicle. There will probably be tender spots on both contacts, so be gentle. Begin to rock both contacts at the same time for about one minute. Then hold for one minute. Repeat this sequence three times. While you're doing the manipulation the tenderness of both contact points should ease up. You may hear digestive gurgles, which indicates that the digestive tract is emptying out. When you break contact, raise both hands directly up off the torso for about one and a half feet before you completely break away from the client's aura. Gentle, graceful manipulations reflect the pureness of the soul, and your client will respond in a positive way to your expression of love.

2. Knee-to-Elbow Contact

Stay on the same side of the table. Place your lower hand above the top of the knee. Place your upper hand on the muscles above the elbow.

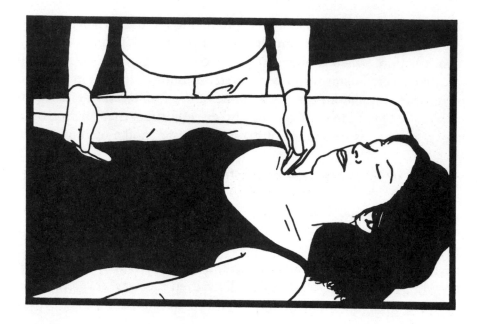

Gently rock both contacts for one minute, then pause for one minute. Repeat the sequence three times. The areas above the knee and elbow on the right side of the body are liver reflexes. The arms are extensions of the torso: by placing your arms next to your torso, you'll see how the elbow corresponds to the liver on the right side and the stomach on the left side. The same relationship holds true when you place the legs alongside the torso. Any sore spots you discover should be relieved by the end of the rocking.

3. Toe-to-Liver Contact

Hold the fire toe with your right hand and place your left hand over the liver. Hold for three minutes. If the foot contact is too far for you to reach, hold the fire finger instead. Repeat on the other foot. Many times the negative pole is where the main blockage is located. By releasing the negative pole the circuit is rejoined.

4. Fire Finger-to-Fire Toe Contact

Hold the fire finger and the fire toe for two minutes. Repeat on the other side. Complete this treatment with the head cradle of your choice to balance the body.

THE KIDNEYS

The kidneys are located between the twelfth thoracic and third lumbar vertebrae. Because the liver takes up such a large area, the right kidney is situated a little lower than the left kidney. The kidneys are about the size of our ears and are filled with thousands of tiny porous vessels that let the blood pass through them.

The primary function of the kidneys is to detoxify the blood. It is the body's liquid filtering system and regulates the concentration and volume of blood in the system. Toxins are removed from the blood and converted into urine, which then moves through a tiny tube called the *ureter* and empties into a holding tank called the *urinary bladder*. When the bladder fills up, the urine is eliminated from the body via the *urethra*. Normally, about 100 quarts of fluid a day are filtered through the kidneys; about two quarts are converted to urine and eliminated.

When the kidneys do not function properly, much of the waste is returned to the blood. This causes the heart to work overtime, as it must beat more strongly to push the sluggish blood throughout the system. The skin is also forced to work harder, as it must produce a larger volume of sweat to assist in the elimination of body fluids.

Eating heavy meals, overeating and diets that consist of large quantities of meat slow down the function of the kidneys. This can lead to high blood pressure, retention of bodily fluids and skin disorders, to name just a few. Consuming a lot of salt clogs the kidneys and makes them work much harder to process the extra fluid the salt retains. Drugs like marijuana, alcohol and amphetamines are major toxins that bombard the kidneys, causing them to be overworked.

To rejuvenate the kidneys and give the system a rest, limit your intake of salt and reduce the amount of food consumed. Stop all drugs, including cigarettes. Fresh carrot and beet juice will help restore proper kidney function. Physical signs that indicate malfunctioning kidneys are: swelling of the ankles, bags under the eyes, dark brown urine, a burning sensation while urinating, water retention throughout the body and chronic skin disorders.

TECHNIQUE TO BALANCE THE KIDNEYS

1. Kidney Flex

Have your client lie on their stomach. Move down to the feet and contact the kidney reflex, midway down the tendon of the big toe, with your thumb. Place your other hand on top of the foot and gently flex the toes downward as you press in with your thumb on the kidney point. This reflex

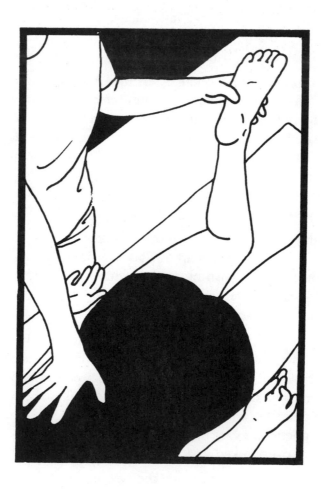

point will probably be a little tender, so be easy. Repeat this flex five times. By the time you are finished the tenderness should subside. Repeat the technique on the other foot.

2. Foot-to-Back Contact

Move to the right side of the table. With your lower hand, bend the knee so the foot is near the buttocks. Place your upper hand over the right kidney area (twelfth thoracic vertebra). Locate and flex the kidney point on the bottom of the foot. Hold both contacts for a few minutes. Move the foot back down to the table and break the above contact. Now repeat on the other side.

3. Sacrum-to-Neck Hold

Return to the right side of the table and place your left hand over the neck and your right hand over the sacrum area of the spine. Hold for one or two minutes, then release by moving both hands straight up for two feet, so that you have completely cleared the person's aura. Many times your client will think you are still holding them after you have finished a manipulation. This is a very powerful and soothing way to conclude a treatment.

DIET

As we constantly seek to replace the energy that is used by our bodies, we are attracted to different kinds of foods and liquids. Foods and liquids are processed by the stomach, assimilated by the intestines, chemically broken down by the liver and the unused remains eliminated by the large intestine. Harmony and balance within are achieved when these four processes function properly without interruption. A malfunction occurs when the natural flow of energy is blocked. This can cause discomfort, pain and eventually disease.

What causes these energy patterns to short-circuit? There are many contributing factors. Someone in my class once asked, "How come everything I like to eat isn't good for me?" Why are we attracted to rich, spicy, processed, chemicalized, denatured foods even though we know they're not good for us? For many people, this food struggle continues throughout their entire lives without them understanding why they crave unhealthy foods.

FIGHTING FOOD CRAVINGS

The answer lies in understanding matter. All physical manifestations of matter find their origins in the mental vibrational field. Mind energy rules physical matter because it is matter in a much purer vibrational form.

Excessive food cravings stem from mental desires being expressed through the senses. The senses help the mind run the body; problems occur when the senses take over and try to satisfy the never-ending mental desires. Why suffer the aftereffects of these uncontrollable impulses? Change the programming of your mind by substituting for your mental tape of constantly craving food one that is empty and desires nothing. Whenever those food cravings besiege you, don't act on them. They should pass in a few minutes (try counting to ten). Try to separate yourself from the mental process. Take a step away from your mind and watch your thoughts in action. When you become a spectator to your thought process, you gain control of your actions because you're no longer compelled to act out each impulse. You can decide consciously which action will be a benefit or a hindrance. If this seems difficult at first, sit down and try the alternate nostril breathing technique (see pages 156–157). This is a wonderful technique that immediately quiets the mind and will assist you in overcoming your mental desires.

After your food urge has subsided, take the time to reaffirm mentally that whenever these food cravings arise, you don't have to act upon them. Don't try to stop them, as resisting these thoughts will only create mental blocks that can carry over into other situations. Instead, let the energy flow freely and through your positive affirmation, the negative imbalanced thoughts that create the food cravings will slowly disappear. Be patient with yourself. At first you may not be able to reverse the pattern 100 percent of the time, but that's all right. In time you'll see that the urges aren't as strong and don't appear with the same frequency. Eventually they'll cease altogether.

THINGS TO REMEMBER WHILE YOU EAT

1. Avoid eating unless you're sitting down. Walking down the street munching on food is a disaster for the entire digestive process.

2. Avoid eating too quickly. If you don't have enough time to complete your meal, eat at a time when you do. Stuffing your face and then running off is disruptive and usually results in poor digestion.

3. Avoid distractions during your meal. Making phone calls or watching TV takes your attention away from what you're doing, causing overeating and slowing down your digestion.

4. Avoid eating when you're angry. It's best to eat at another time, because your food can't be thoroughly digested when anger or other negative emotions are present.

5. Stop eating when you feel full. Overeating clogs and overworks all your digestive organs. Sometimes the food just sits along the digestive tract because you shoveled in twice the amount your body can digest effectively. This excess food will then ferment, producing gas which can cause pain if not released.

6. Eat only when you're hungry and drink only when you're thirsty. Eating when you're thirsty and drinking when you're hungry will disrupt your system and cause problems later on.

7. Bless your food before eating it. Offering the food to the Creator changes its vibration and makes it easier to digest. This is especially true when eating out in restaurants, because you don't know the state of mind of the chef or food server. If the chef is upset at something while preparing your food, those vibrations will be transmitted into the food, making it more difficult to digest. Likewise, if the food server is being hassled, your lunch or dinner will arrive containing those uptight feelings and will be difficult to digest properly. Blessing the food removes such negativity and makes for a better meal.

Proper food selection is an individual decision which we learn through trial and error. The thing to remember is that the right food for one individual isn't always right for another. There are no set rules to conform to. Your age, constitution, capability to digest and assimilate and temperament are all contributing factors in determining what foods are best suited for you. By acknowledging these factors, you can establish a well-balanced eating pattern. It's up to you to take the time to figure out what's best for you. No one else can. It's your life and you must make your own choices.

ABOUT MEALS

1. Simple meals are best suited for digestion. Eating a wide variety of foods at one sitting confuses the enzyme-producing organs, which then produce the wrong kinds or amounts of digestive juices.

2. All solid food should be well chewed and insalivated. We often forget that digestion begins in the mouth. Most people don't chew their food enough, and it enters the stomach in lumps. Then it takes a long time for the food to be broken down into a state suitable for the duodenum.

3. Eat your meal slowly. When you eat fast, you aren't conscious of the amount of food you consume at each sitting. Slowing down the process brings that awareness back and will help you stop overeating.

4. Too many spices at one meal can be an irritant.

5. Liquifying solid foods in a blender confuses the digestive organs and they don't respond with the proper enzymic production.

TASTE

Ayurvedic medicine has developed a wonderful system which helps us understand how different foods affect the body, depending on their taste. This enables the Ayurvedic physican to establish a food guideline to suit the individual needs of each patient. According to this system, all tastes fall into six categories which can be translated as: bitter, tart, sour, salty, sweet and strong. The following chart describes them and shows their relationship to the elements:

		RELATIONSHIP TO ELEMENTS	
TASTE	DESCRIPTION	INCREASE	DECREASE
Bitter	Unpleasant, acid, contracting	Air	Earth/Fire
Tart	Contracts tissues and organs	Air	Earth/Fire
Sour	Sharp, acid fermented, unpleasant, stinging	Fire/Earth	Air
Salty	Sharp, tangy	Fire/Earth	Air
Sweet	Pleasant, sugary	Earth	Fire/Air
Strong	Sharp, penetrating, biting	Fire/Air	Earth

How does this translate into information you can use? *Bitter* foods make a person light and mobile. They lighten the load and are recommended for overweight, lethargic people who have a difficult time being motivated and have a tendency to accumulate things. Conversely, the person who can create wonderful ideas but can't manifest them on the physical plane, is always up in the air, is very mental and can't seem to stay grounded, should stay away from bitter foods because they increase their tendency toward airiness.

Tart foods contract tissues and organs, causing a drying effect on the body. They are recommended for people who are emotional all the time, have water retention in the body, loose bowel movements or diarrhea, a constant runny nose, too much mucus in their system and a general feeling of always being "watered down." On the other hand, people who are constipated, have rigid, fixed ideas and are unwilling to yield on any position in life should stay away from tart foods or their condition will worsen.

Sour foods stimulate digestion and are recommended for people who are cold all the time or have poor circulation and need extra warmth. They stimulate the digestive process and help maintain an even energy flow. Sour foods stimulate the appetite, increase the secretion of digestive juices and air those who are finicky eaters. Anyone who needs a mental boost will benefit from sour foods because they increase the oxidation process, which allows the brain to better utilize the amount of oxygen in the blood. Conversely, too much sour food can cause heartburn and oversecretion of acid in the stomach, which can cause ulcers. A person who is hot-headed might become irritated even easier by consuming a lot of sour foods. Sour foods can also increase your thirst and should be avoided by people who have a problem with water retention.

Salty foods aid digestion and have the ability to increase body heat. They also increase the quality of food by improving its general taste. Salty foods promote the secretion of saliva, which is the first part of the digestive process. In times of sickness, salty foods help flush the system because they make you want to increase your liquid consumption. If someone has experienced a great water loss from sickness or diarrhea, it's important to replace the salt level in the body before dehydration sets in. The same holds true when any strenuous physical activity occurs and the water level of the body is reduced rapidly.

However, too much salt in the body can cause high blood pressure, which makes the heart work harder to do its job. Also, too much salt causes the body to retain a high level of water, which can cause the kidneys to work overtime processing it. Many skin disorders are caused when the kidneys can't function properly due to overwork. People who are overly emotional should watch their intake of salty foods closely. Too much water in the system can affect your equilibrium and make you feel as though you are about to float away.

Naturally *Sweet* foods nourish and soothe the body. They supply lots of energy that can be used now or stored for later. They give the body strength and are needed to help rebuild and repair old, used tissues. People who are nervous, anxious and can't seem to get a grip on their overstimulated minds will benefit from sweet foods because these will bring them down to earth. On the other hand, those who move slowly, lack motivation in life, are overweight and can't seem to fall asleep at night should stay away from sweet foods. Light, bitter foods will give these people a little more mobility and help counteract their lethargic attitude.

Strong foods are a digestive aid and help in the assimilation of food. They are recommended for people with digestive troubles. Those who often have a sour stomach will benefit from strong foods. They increase heat in the body and improve circulation, which cleanses the body by speeding up the metabolism and burning off accumulated wastes. Strong foods help the skin eliminate wastes as well. They can help clear up a constant runny nose. Conversely, aggressive individuals may become more aggressive if they consume strong foods, so they should limit their intake of these foods.

The following list classifies some common foods according to their taste:

BITTER	TART	SOUR	SALTY	SWEET	STRONG
carrots	golden seal	yogurt	salt	milk	red pepper
tumeric	butter	cheese	sea salt	sugar	garlic
sesame	eggs	citrus	soy sauce	rice	onion
cinnamon	soy beans	fruits	kelp	wheat	ginger
	kidney beans			licorice	chili
	broccoli			honey	mustard
	cabbage			maple	radish
	cauliflower			syrup	clove
				beets	

IS IT ORGANIC?

Finding organic foods can be difficult. There are few stores that can get certified organic products, especially if you live in a rural community. Natural food stores usually carry a full line of unprocessed whole foods; however, these foods are not always organic.

In organic growing, the soil contains no pesticides, artificial fertilizers or herbicides. The crop is not sprayed at any time during its growing process, and the result is a pure, high-quality food, rich in nutrients and life force. Organic foods look different, smell different, and taste different from processed foods. Most of the products in the major food-chain stores are processed, chemicalized, artifically colored and flavored denatured foods with limited nutritional value. The food in these stores looks good and can remain on the shelves for a long period of time without spoiling, but the chemicals in them that make this possible have made the food nutritionally worthless. Certain food colorings in use on the market have even caused cancer in laboratory animals. The chemical companies have conducted their own tests, with positive results. The F.D.A. has had these results for a number of years, so the fact that they have not removed these cancer-causing colorings from all food is outrageous. Obviously, the food coloring industry has been lobbying hard for the F.D.A. to take no action, because this is a 30-billion-dollar-a-year industry and has a lot of clout. Money talks. As consumers, we can refuse to purchase these products. If you don't want to be poisoned and care about your health, read all the labels on the foods you purchase and select only the ones that are unprocessed and, if possible, certifiably organic.

Unfortunately, there is no national agency that certifies farms as organic. It is up to your local health-food stores to verify whether or not the products that are claimed to be organic really are. Quite often the distributors of organic foods check out the growers themselves and report their findings to the local health-food stores. There is a lot of trust among the distributors and health-food stores when it comes to organic products because no one can really say for sure whether a product was grown chemically free. At best, this situation leaves a lot of questions unanswered.

SEASONAL EFFECTS ON DIET

Living in harmony with our environment demands that we take note of the environmental changes occurring throughout the year. As the seasons come and go, they have certain qualities that affect us. For example, in the springtime, there is no set weather pattern. Many different kinds of weather occur during this season, so it's hard to know just what to do. Adjusting to the many different patterns that affect your area is a good idea. But as spring moves on, the weather usually warms up and showers make planting possible. It is a time of growth when life just bursts through after the long winter. Eating protein foods will help this new growth sprout through you.

In the summertime it can be very warm, even hot. Under such conditions, eating spicy foods that can increase body heat is not recommended.

Autumn is harvest time. The heat of summer has dissipated and the weather becomes cooler and drier. Foods that are bitter, dry and tart, like broccoli, cabbage, celery, beans and sesame seeds, should be consumed in limited quantities because they increase dryness in the body. Leafy vegetables, melons, squash, honey and milk all contain lots of water and are good to eat because they counteract the dryness of the autumn season.

After the harvest it becomes cold and wet as winter sets in. There is usually less activity because we spend more time indoors avoiding the harsh climate. Fruits, cooling foods and sweets should not be consumed in large quantities because, together with the sedentary routines of winter, they can cause weight increases. Heat-producing foods like grains and spices are recommended instead to help burn off the coldness and excess weight.

As the seasons change there's usually a transition period during which we have not quite left one season but we're not yet into the other. During this time, you may have a tendency to come down with a cold or the flu because you haven't adjusted to the new season and your body rhythm is out of balance. Short periods of fasting are a wonderful natural way to ease the transition and give your digestive system a rest.

FOOD COMBINATIONS

If you want food to be digested properly by your digestive system, understanding what happens to food as it's being digested will help you make the right food choices when you eat.

The following food combinations should be avoided because they slow down the digestive process:

1. Starches and Proteins

When starches like potatoes, wheat, rice, corn, oats, etc., are combined with proteins like meats or beans, digestion is slowed because both types of food require different types of enzymes for proper digestion. The starches are digested by the alkaline enzymes found in the mouth and small intestine. The proteins are digested by the acid enzymes found in the stomach. The acid enzymes of the stomach destroy the alkaline enzymes from the mouth that have already begun to break down the starches. So the digestion of starches is greatly slowed, which can cause indigestion. Please note: When whole foods containing both starches and proteins are consumed by themselves, the starch portion is broken down in the stomach through the action of *ptylin*, the enzyme secreted in the mouth. Once this process is almost complete, the stomach secretes its enzymes and the acid begins to break down the protein.

2. Starches and Acidic Foods

The acid found in fruits like oranges, lemons, limes, grapefruit, etc., will destroy the alkaline enzymes needed to properly digest starches. The starches will then ferment, causing excess gas and indigestion.

3. Starches and Sugars

When starches are consumed with sugars, the sugar stops the secretion of the alkaline enzymes needed to digest the starches, resulting in their fermentation. The constant consumption of cakes, donuts and pastries will lead to indigestion and other digestive difficulties.

4. Proteins and Acidic Foods

When acidic foods like citrus fruits, tomatoes and vinegar are consumed with proteins, they can stop the flow of digestive enzymes in the stomach and prevent the proteins from being digested.

5. Proteins

Every protein has its own specific digestive enzyme that is needed for proper digestion. If you consume more than one protein at a time, it quickly becomes difficult for your body to digest the other proteins.

6. Proteins and Fats

When fats like margarine, cooking oils, etc., are eaten with proteins like nuts, meats, eggs, etc., the fats stop the flow of enzymes that digest the proteins, causing many problems with digestion.

7. Proteins and Sugars

Sugars of any kind will slow down the flow of enzymes that digest proteins. The proteins will be digested first and the sugars will wait until the proteins move along before they can be digested.

The following is a list of food combinations that will ensure proper digestion and assimilation:

1. Vegetables and proteins combine well together.
2. Vegetables and starches combine well together.
3. Sweet fruits like bananas, dates, dried fruit, etc., are best eaten alone.
4. Fruits that contain a high level of acid, like oranges, limes, lemons, etc., are best eaten alone.
5. Combining partially acidic fruits like apricots, berries, plums, etc., with sweet fruits is all right.
6. Any type of melon is best consumed by itself.

Food selection and combination is an individual choice. Of course it's best to make the right decisions and avoid indigestion; however, if you do suffer from any digestive difficulties you should start watching the types of food you eat at each meal and notice the reaction your body has to the different food selections you make. The above guideline is only a beginning in discovering what to eat to avoid indigestion. And remember, you choose what you eat, so it's up to you to think about your food selection and make the right choices.

THINGS TO REMEMBER WHILE EATING

1. Food is digested in layers. The first thing eaten will be the first thing digested.

2. Don't be fooled by processed or chemicalized food. They can trick you into overeating because they're easy to eat and taste so good. These foods

are usually eaten quickly, with little regard for caloric intake. As a result, the body receives an abundant supply of calories without getting any nutritional value. Stopping this vicious cycle is the beginning of new eating habits centered around moderation.

3. It's very important that your food be as fresh as possible. For many years I thought that raw sunflower seeds naturally tasted a little bitter. When I finally ate some that were really fresh, I couldn't believe the difference! Wheat germ is another product that goes bad quickly. It must be eaten within a few days after being hulled or it will spoil, regardless of the packaging.

4. As you see, smell and taste your food, the body begins to secrete digestive enzymes. If the food is disguised with different sauces, perservatives and chemicals, your digestive system doesn't know how to react. This causes poor digestion. When this pattern is repeated over a long period of time, diseases can set in, and then you wonder how you got sick.

5. If you aren't hungry, or food doesn't taste good to you, your digestive juices won't flow properly and your food will be poorly digested.

If you really want your food to be efficiently utilized without any residues left behind, you must start to think about your eating patterns. You have been led to believe that diet has nothing to do with the diseases of the body. The prevailing opinion has been that all you have to do is take a pill when you get sick and everything will be okay. Are we really that naive? We are the most technologically advanced society in the history of this planet, but we have paid the price for this by losing touch with, and respect for, nature and the naturally healthy state of our bodies. We're bombarded daily with the message "buy, buy, buy." You can't go anywhere without being subjected to massive media stimulation, exhorting you to do this and buy that or your life will be worthless. We're a nation of consumers, so when we get sick we want to buy a pill to fix that too.

It's up to you to ignore these demands and seek a balance within yourself. Only then can you be content and live peacefully and sensibly.

We are what we eat. Think about what *you* eat, when you eat it. Eat with love and stop eating when you're full. A balanced diet of 60 percent grains, 20 to 30 percent fresh fruits and vegetables, 5 percent nuts and seeds and 5 percent fat will enable you to maintain a healthy body and keep all your bodily systems working efficiently.

CHAKRA BALANCING

The *chakras* are swirls of esoteric energy. There are seven chakras in the body, located along the spine. Just as the axis through the north and south poles maintains the balance of energy of planet Earth, the body has a similar axis, with the *crown chakra* at the top of the head and the *root chakra* at the base of the spine. All energies, all powers, all experiences are stored between these two poles.

When a child is created in its mother's womb, the crown chakra in the head is formed first. The nerves that branch out from the brain form the spinal column and the other chakras. Each chakra has an identifying sound, color, element, quality and shape.

As each chakra is formed, it takes the divine energy it needs. This is not to say that by the time the last chakra is formed it is receiving the leftover energy from the other chakras. Each chakra is different, and needs a different energy in its formation. There is always enough energy for the formation of them all.

KUNDALINI

This energy is called *Kundalini* and lies dormant in the root chakra after its descent down the spine. Kundalini is the manifestation of God-power in the human being, a spiritual force that is the essence of all life. When this energy is reawakened, it travels up the spine, going through each chakra, cleansing it along the way. When if completes its ascent and merges in the crown chakra, a state of complete oneness with all creation, or God consciousness, is achieved.

However, if a person is not ready to receive such a blast of energy, it can burn out their nervous system, in much the same way as a 50-watt bulb would explode if it were screwed into a socket for 1,000,000 watts. It is most important to find a teacher who knows exactly the right moment to reawaken this energy within you, or else you may run the risk of becoming that 50-watt bulb. When you are ready, a true teacher will manifest.

THE SEVEN CHAKRAS

The *first chakra* is located at the base of the spine and is called the *root chakra,* or *Muladhara.*

Color:	red	Element:	Earth
Shape:	square	Sound:	*lam*
Quality:	*tamas*	Body Function:	elimination of solids
Body Part:	rectum, bowels, colon, bladder	Emotion:	fear

Most of your material concerns and survival needs are stored here. Anything to do with the physical plane, touch, mental anxiety or nervousness finds its center here.

The *second chakra* is located between the navel and the genitals. It is called *Svadhishthana.*

Color:	orange	Element:	Water
Shape:	crescent moon	Sound:	*vam*
Quality:	*rajas*	Body Function:	sexual energy
Body Part:	reproductive organs, lymph, blood, urine, semen	Emotion:	attachment

Your creativity and desire are centered here. The drive to maintain the species, sensuality, lust, greed, and along with the root chakra, material needs, can be found here.

The *third chakra* is located just above the navel. It is called *Manipura.*

Color:	yellow	Element:	Fire
Shape:	triangle turned down	Sound:	*ram*
		Body Function:	digestion and assimilation
Quality:	*rajas*		
Body Part:	stomach, liver, spleen, gall bladder	Emotion:	anger

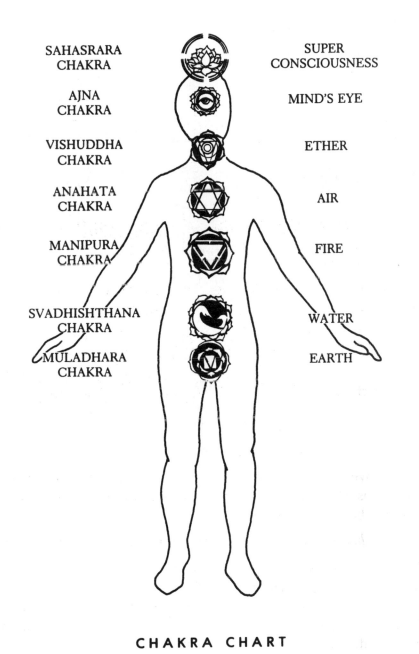

SAHASRARA
CHAKRA

AJNA
CHAKRA

VISHUDDHA
CHAKRA

ANAHATA
CHAKRA

MANIPURA
CHAKRA

SVADHISHTHANA
CHAKRA

MULADHARA
CHAKRA

SUPER
CONSCIOUSNESS

MIND'S EYE

ETHER

AIR

FIRE

WATER

EARTH

CHAKRA CHART

Willpower, how you view yourself and whether you trust your inner voices are all centered here, as well as the process of assimilating food for your body.

The *fourth chakra* is located in the chest. It is called the *heart chakra* or *Anahata.*

Color:	green	Element:	Air
Shape:	hexagon, reversed triangles	Sound:	*yam*
		Body Function:	distribution of air through-
Quality:	*sattva*		out the body
Body Part:	heart and lungs		
		Emotion:	grief

The love you feel for all things and the emotions that go along with that love are stored here. Your life energy is processed through the breath and begins here. Your compassion and self-expression also come from this chakra.

The *fifth chakra* is located in the throat. It is called *Vishudda.*

Color:	blue	Element:	Ether
Shape:	circle	Sound:	*ham*
Quality:	*sattva*	Body Function:	speech and
Body Part:	throat, thyroid and parathyroid		regulation of metabolism

The throat chakra is the bridge from your higher being to your lower being. All energy going up and down passes through the throat center. Speech, self-expression and communication are all centered here.

The *sixth chakra* is located between the eyebrows. It is called *Ajna,* or third eye.

Color:	indigo	Sound:	*aum*
Shape:	round	Body Function:	mind's eye
Quality:	*sattva*		

The third eye is the center of intuition, perception, devotion and higher awareness. It is the entrance to the divine kingdom within.

The *seventh chakra* is located at the top of the head. It is called the *crown chakra* or *Sahasrara.*

Color:	violet	Sound:	*om*

It is the seat of cosmic consciousness, or God-realization.

TECHNIQUE FOR CHAKRA BALANCING

It is important to think in terms of balance, not opening. Each chakra has much energy that has accumulated from both past and present experiences; without direct supervision from a true spiritual master you don't want to open any chakra. If the chakra has too much or too little energy, you merely want to bring its rate of vibration back to normal.

While balancing the chakras, you can experiment by visualizing the color of each chakra. A good way to remember the color sequence is to remember the name "Roy G. Biv." Each letter stands for a different color, starting with the root chakra: Red, Orange, Yellow, Green, Blue, Indigo, Violet.

1. Have your client lie on their stomach. Remove all articles of clothing, such as belts, that might get in the way. Move to the right side of the table and place your left hand gently on the back of the neck. Place your right

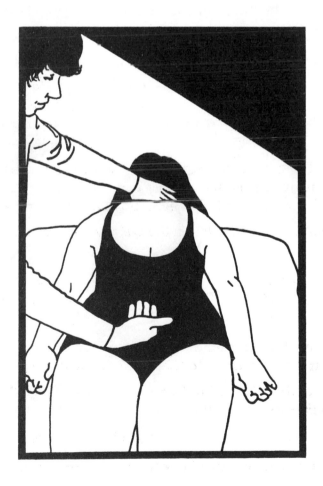

hand, with palm facing up, on the *coccyx* (tail bone), midway down the buttocks. Hold gently for three to four minutes, with your fingers pointing straight up toward the top of the spine. Then move your right hand (palm down) so that it rests horizontally across the same area, gently rocking for about one minute. Then hold gently for one minute. For all other contacts the palm lies flat on the contact point.

2. Move your right hand up to the sacrum, on the second chakra, and repeat the process.

3. Move your right hand up to the fire center, behind the navel center, and repeat the process.

4. Move your right hand up to the shoulder blades, on the fourth chakra, and repeat the process.

5. When you move to the throat, switch hands, so that now the right hand is behind the neck.

6. Gently place the thumb of your left hand on your client's third eye and hold gently.

7. Move the thumb of your left hand to the crown chakra and hold gently.

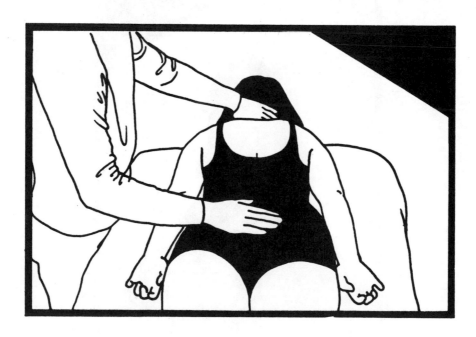

This completes the sequence. You will notice that your client becomes quiet and will sometimes go to sleep during this treatment. Be very quiet during this session and give the person a chance to relax. This is very calming and balancing to the entire system. It is especially good for headaches, tension, stress, nervousness and general disharmony.

THE FIVE-POINTED STAR

The five-pointed star is a representation in the body of the law, "As above, so below." If the bottom of a structure is weak, so must the top be weak. What happens to one directly affects the other.

If we look at the torso minus the arms and legs, we find that tension in the shoulders corresponds to tension in the hips. By working with the diagonal currents of the torso, we can bring great relief from tension and soreness to both the shoulders and the hips. The diagonal currents represent the figure eight of energy within the body. They are said to be part of the chemistry of creation affecting each cell in all living things. All the internal organs—heart, lungs, kidneys, intestines, stomach, liver, bladder and reproductive system—will benefit from having the torso currents re-established in their natural patterns.

The two pelvic points of the star are where sensory tension and emotional frustration accumulate. The pelvis is the negative pole of the torso, and the body's energy has a tendency to get stuck there. This stops its natural flow back upwards. Therefore, the throat, shoulders and neck have their reflex points at the hips. By releasing the tension there, harmony is restored.

TECHNIQUE FOR THE FIVE-POINTED STAR

Have your client lie on their back and move to the left side of the table. Place your right hand on your client's left shoulder and your left hand on their left hip. Rock for one minute, then pause for 30 seconds. Repeat three times. Now move your right hand to their right shoulder (keep your left hand on your client's left hip) and repeat the rock-and-pause sequence three times. Slowly lift both hands straight up off the torso and break contact. Move to the right side of the table. Place your left hand on your client's left shoulder and your right hand on their right hip. Repeat the rock-and-pause sequence three times. Move your left hand to your client's right shoulder and repeat the rock-and-pause sequence three times. Keep your right hand on the right hip and place the air finger of your left hand on your client's chin. Hold for one minute. Remember to hold gently for 30 seconds between all rocks. This is the time when the body will have most of its major releases.

THE NECK

Everyone has suffered from a sore throat or pain in the neck some time in their lives. It's usually the first sign of a cold or an indication that the person is having difficulty in expressing their true feelings. This treatment will bring relief from the physical symptoms of a sore throat or any pain in the neck, including muscle spasms or misplaced vertebrae. The neck is not twisted or snapped during this treatment. Realignment occurs in a gentle way as the energy patterns are re-established.

TECHNIQUE TO BALANCE THE NECK

1. Throat and Neck Points

Have your client lie on their back. Face your client's head. Place your left fire finger at the base of the throat along the left side of the adam's apple. Locate any sore spot there. Place your right air finger at the base of the neck by the spinal column on the right side. Locate any sore spot there. Alternately wiggle each contact for about 15 seconds, then pause for about 30 seconds. Repeat three times. Move each contact up to the middle of the throat and repeat the sequence, then move up to the top of the throat and repeat it again. Reverse your hands and repeat the entire sequence on the other side. This series of contacts will relieve tenderness in the throat and neck.

2. Pubic Bone-to-Chin Bone Contact

Move to the right side of the table. Place the fire finger of your right hand on the soft tissue just above the center of the pubic bone. Be sure to inform your client where this contact will be before you make it, as it is a sensitive area. Place the air finger of your left hand on the center of the chin. Hold this contact for about two minutes. The pubic and chin bones are opposite ends of the same energy field. This contact will send energy through the neck and clear any blockage.

3. Thumb-to-Big Toe Contact

The first sections of the thumb and big toe both reflex to the neck area. With the ether and air fingers of both hands contact the first sections of the big toe and thumb. This contact should bring about a release in the neck area. Hold and stimulate each contact for about one minute. Go to the other side of the table and repeat the contact on that side.

4. Big Toe Adjustment

This powerful adjustment of the big toe can have wonderful results. Once a student came to class after being in a car accident in which she suffered a whiplash. Her neck was in a brace and she was in a lot of pain. She had been to a chiropractor but was too sore to receive an adjustment. She should have been in bed resting but decided to come to class, hoping for some support and relief. It just so happened that I was demonstrating the neck treatment that day and I worked on her. Nothing I did was helping until the big toe adjustment. After the big toe adjustment, all the vertebrae in her neck self-adjusted and she was able to take off her neck brace. Most of her pain subsided. The reason this works so well is that the base of the

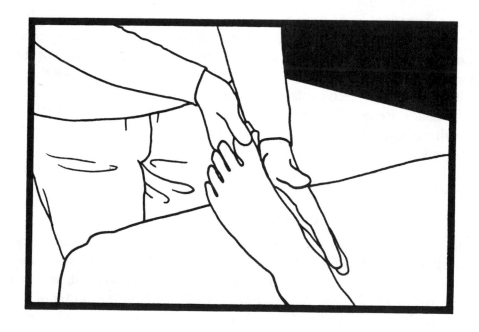

big toe reflexes directly to the atlas of the spine. Once the base of the joint clicks in, relief is instant.

Move down to the feet. On the right side (the client's left foot), hold the big toe back as far as it will comfortably go. With the fleshy part of the base of your thumb, firmly slap the base of the joint of the big toe. There should be a clicking sound as the joint adjusts. If it doesn't work the first time, repeat three or four times. Don't try this adjustment on someone who has gout or arthritis. It is a deeply moving manipulation and can be very powerful in bringing dramatic relief. Repeat on the other foot if the first side doesn't click in. If it does, it isn't necessary to do the other foot.

5. Hand-to-Opposite Foot Hold

Move to the right side of the table. With your left hand, hold your client's right hand. Now with your right hand, reach over and hold your client's left foot. Hold for one to two minutes, then gently release. Now move to the other side of the table and with your right hand, hold your client's left hand. Then with your left hand, reach over and hold your client's right foot for about two minutes, then release.

THE CHAIR TREATMENT

The Chair Treatment is simple, effective and easy to do. All you need is a chair and someone who has a headache, tight shoulders or a pain in their back. Unlike other treatments, for which you need a table, oil, sheets, an hour and a half and soothing background music, the Chair Treatment can bring relief in from ten to fifteen minutes. It is the "quick fix" society is always looking for. People want things in a hurry, including relief from pain. This treatment fulfills that desire, as it quickly relieves tension in the upper half of the body. It's the perfect treatment for people who sit all day at work. I have used this treatment in restaurants, train stations, on boats, in offices, at parks and family gatherings. People love it.

TECHNIQUE FOR THE CHAIR TREATMENT:

Have your client sit in a chair straddle fashion.

1. Head Hold

Stand behind the client, then move to the left so you are facing their ear. Place your right hand behind the neck and your left hand on the forehead above the eyebrows. Hold for one minute. This will balance the central nervous system and bring immediate relief from a headache.

2. Shoulder Rub

Stand behind your client. Place both hands on your client's shoulders (trapezius muscle). Using all your fingers, knead the entire trapezius muscle. Check with your client to make sure you aren't hurting them. Also rub the arms down to the elbows. Rub for three to five minutes. This move always feels great. It breaks up shoulder tension, which is a common complaint.

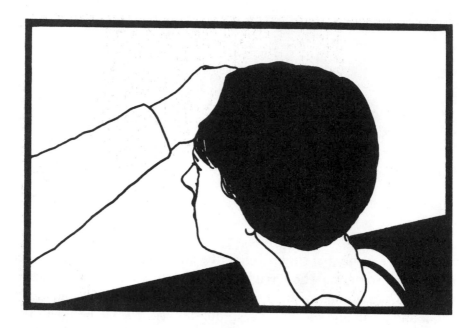

3. Spinal Flex

Place your thumbs on either side of the spine at the shoulders. Step by step, vertebra by vertebra, move down the spine to the sacrum, stimulating each contact with a wiggle. This will help break up gas pockets that develop in these muscles due to poor digestion. Repeat three times.

4. Scapula Release

Bend the elbow and place the forearm and hand in a horizontal position behind the back. You will notice that the scapula is protruding due to the position of the arm. Place one hand on the front side of the shoulder; with your other hand make contact under the scapula, starting at the bottom. You can use your fingers or thumb to make a stimulating contact as you slowly work your way up the entire scapula. You will notice that the higher you get along the scapula, the more tension you will find. Be gentle and don't force it. For people who are very tight here, just a little release will bring wonderful relief. People who receive the most benefit are those with breathing difficulties and those who hold tension in this area.

5. Tapotement

In a rhythmic motion, with palms open and fingers closed, alternately stimulate the trapezius muscle and the midback with the tips of your little fingers. Pause after two minutes and repeat three times. This move is very stimulating and disperses blocked energy.

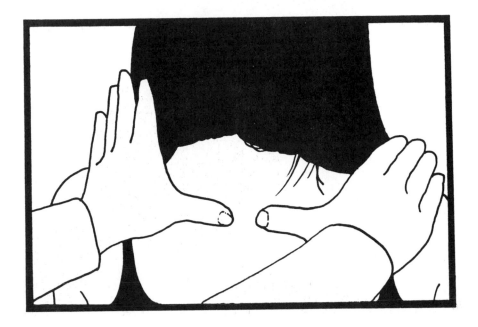

6. Neck Rub

Place one hand on the forehead and the other behind the neck, the same position as in the Head Hold. With the thumb of the hand on the neck contact, begin to rub the neck, starting at the base of the skull along the occipital ridge. Move out toward the ear, down along the outside neck to the shoulders, then back to the spine and up to where you started. Repeat five times on either side. This will ease tension in the neck and prevent headaches.

7. Brush Off

Place both hands on top of the head; using a slow, easy motion, brush the energy off the body as you move down to the waist. Repeat three to four times. This will clear the person's aura of any excess energy and conclude the treatment.

THE ARMS AND HANDS

You would really be lost without your hands. There is hardly any activity you engage in during your life that doesn't include the use of your hands, yet they often go unnoticed for months at a time. During your stay in your mother's womb, your hands were crossed over your heart; they have absorbed the heart's energy and maintain that special quality.

The arms are extensions of your torso, and give you the freedom of expressing your thoughts. They also maintain circulatory reflexes.

TECHNIQUE FOR THE ARMS AND HANDS

1. Wrist Flip

Bend the arm at the elbow, so the hand is upright. Place both thumbs behind your client's wrist. Place your other four fingers symmetrically down from the wrist joint, then flip the wrist back and forth ten times.

2. Wrist Rotation

Hold your client's wrist with one hand; with the other hand hold the thumb or fingers and rotate the wrist ten times in each direction.

3. Inner Forearm-to-Thumb Web Contact

With your outer hand contact the thumb web point between thumb and index finger (air finger on top and ether finger on the palm side). With your inner hand contact the inner forearm point. From the crease of the elbow, go down one inch along the inside forearm, then one inch toward the center of the arm. This is the inside forearm contact. It reflexes to the heart. Alternately stimulate the thumb web point and the inner forearm point for about 30 seconds each. Then pause for about ten seconds. Repeat three times.

4. Outer Arms-to-Torso Contact

From the outer elbow crease, come down one inch, then move in one inch to the outer arm contact; this reflexes to the lungs. Let your client's hand rest on your torso. Then with your other hand contact the torso on the same line. Alternately stimulate each contact for about 30 seconds. The torso stimulation is an upward movement using the air, fire and water fingers. The right side torso contact is the liver. The left side torso contact is the spleen.

5. Finger Strokes

Stroke the tendons of each finger on the back of your client's hand. Rotate

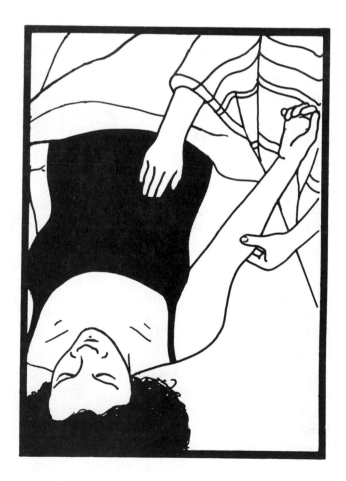

each finger ten times in both directions. With your inside hand hold the thumb with your ether, air and fire fingers. Contact the arm just below the wrist and with both hands give a gentle tug in opposite directions. Move to the contact just below the elbow, then below the shoulder, and give a gentle tug at each contact. Repeat with each finger.

HAND CHART

FIRE ELEMENT

AIR ELEMENT

WATER ELEMENT

MOUND OF VENUS

THE HAND CHART

The information from the Hand Chart provides us with an instant Polarity treatment that can be applied anywhere, at any time, whenever the need arises. The zodiac and the five elements of Ether, Air, Fire, Water and Earth have a direct relationship. Each zodiacal sign corresponds to a different part of the body. Understanding this relationship is the secret of these mini-treatments.

The Earth Element is represented by the little finger of the hand. The three sections between the joints of the finger correspond to the three Earth zodiacal signs: Taurus, Virgo and Capricorn. Taurus corresponds to the top digit of the earth finger. Taurus is the Bull, and like the bull, a person born under this sign is usually stubborn and set in their ways, with an unwillingness to make changes in their daily routines. The body part represented by Taurus is the neck.

HAND TREATMENT

Anyone having difficulties with their throat or neck will benefit from this treatment. Have the person sit down. Place your left hand on the neck or throat and with your right hand, squeeze the sides of the top section of their earth finger for about 15 seconds. Then pause for about one minute and repeat the sequence five times. Then hold both contacts gently for three minutes. Usually the section that corresponds to the ailing body part will be a little sore when squeezed. By the time you're finished with the treatment, there shouldn't be any pain. Sensitive people will feel the energy block loosen up, and their condition should improve. Throughout the treatment have your client close their eyes and breathe deeply. This will help facilitate the release of the energy block and involve the person in their own healing process.

To confirm that what you are doing is correct, check all the other sections of the fingers with a healthy squeeze. The only soreness you find should relate to the body part in question; all other sections should not hurt. If another section is tender, it's probably because of a dormant energy block that has not yet manifested, or it could be due to the person's sun sign. The sun sigh (birth sign) indicates a potential weak point in the corresponding body part. If these factors don't apply and there is no other apparent explanation, don't worry about it. The person can probably still use the treatment, and that is the most important thing to remember. Do the work and don't be concerned with explaining it or with the results. The treatment is the same for all the sections of the fingers.

The following chart breaks down the correspondences so that they can be easily understood and applied:

ELEMENT	FINGER	ZODIACAL SIGN	BODY PART	LOCATION
Earth	Little	Taurus	Neck, Throat	Top Section
Earth	Little	Virgo	Bowels	Middle Section
Earth	Little	Capricorn	Knees	Bottom Section
Water	Ring	Cancer	Breast	Top Section
Water	Ring	Scorpio	Genitals	Middle Section
Water	Ring	Pisces	Feet	Bottom Section
Fire	Middle	Aries	Head, Eyes	Top Section
Fire	Middle	Leo	Solar plexus	Middle Section
Fire	Middle	Sagittarius	Thighs	Bottom Section
Air	Pointer	Gemini	Shoulders	Top Section
Air	Pointer	Libra	Kidneys	Middle Section
Air	Pointer	Aquarius	Ankles	Bottom Section
Ether	Thumb	No Sign	Head	Top Section
Ether	Thumb	No Sign	Neck	Bottom Section
Ether	Thumb	No Sign	Back	Bone of Thumb

So wherever you are, whatever you're doing, if someone injures themselves, has a sprain, muscle spasms, headaches, etc., applying this information will provide a powerful instant treatment that helps bring quick relief.

THE BACK

It's no wonder that so many people in our society complain of some form of back pain. Your back reflects the general state of your well-being. When things in your life are in a state of disharmony, your body reacts with pain. The pain is a signal that something is wrong and that a change in your way of life is necessary.

The spine is to the body what its axis is to the planet Earth. Each one represents the core energy of its own organism, and the slightest tilt from center has a great effect upon the whole.

Each vertebra along the spinal column has a specific reflex to all the organs and muscles of the body. Soreness along any vertebra indicates energy blocks. Quite often there are too many incoming impulses, causing the outward expression to slow down or cease. In the case of a chronic disorder, look at the chakra that houses the sore vertebra for some clue to the problem. In any event, a back session will bring relief to most ailments and restore the proper energy channels, allowing everything to circulate, like air in a well-vented house.

As a rule, the back is the last part of the body we work on during the general session. We have better results with the back once the entire body is relaxed, and the energy balancing will last longer.

TECHNIQUE TO BALANCE THE BACK

1. Sacrum Rock

Have your client lie on their stomach. Move to the right side of the table. Place your left hand over your client's neck and your right hand, slightly cupped, over their *coccyx* (tail bone). Rock with your right hand for 30 seconds, then hold lightly for 30 seconds. Your left hand should remain lightly in place throughout this technique. Repeat three times.

This contact will help the lower back and release any tension in the hips. Remember to tell your client to move their head to the other side slowly should any neck strain occur.

2. Opposite Shoulder-to-Hip Rock

Place your left hand on your client's left shoulder and your right hand on their right hip. Alternately rock each contact for 30 seconds and hold lightly for 30 seconds. Repeat three times, then switch hands and treat the opposite side.

3. Spinal Walk

Place the ether and air fingers of your left hand on either side of the top cervical vertebra. Place the ether and air fingers of your right hand alongside the coccyx vertebra. Your fingers should be on the muscles directly alongside the spine, not on the spine itself. Slowly rock your right hand, using medium pressure, while moving up the spine vertebra by vertebra. With your left hand continue holding the contact above gently. This will release most energy blocks along the spine. Repeat a second time.

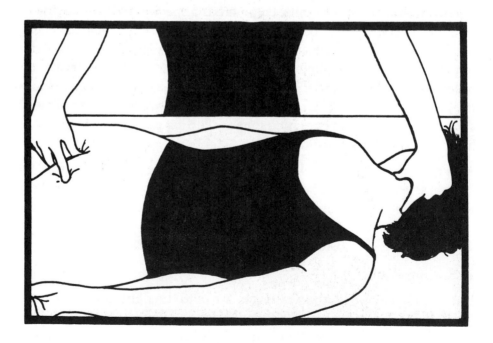

If you find a sore spot, hold gently and channel energy. Then move your left hand down, so that both hands are contacted just above and below the sore vertebra. Now you can create a diagonal current through the sore vertebra by releasing the ether finger of one hand and the air finger of the other hand. Reverse and repeat five times. This will release specific tension in the vertebrae. The back is symmetrical, so the coccyx and cervical vertebrae affect each other. As above, so below.

Now with your left hand, hold the sore vertebra. Bend your client's knee so that the foot rises up, then contact the appropriate point on the arch of the foot in relation to the sore vertebra. This is a very powerful contact which often breaks through any blocked energy.

4. Scapula Release

Bend your client's elbow, placing their forearm and hand behind their back. This will expose their scapula (shoulder blade). Place your upper hand underneath their shoulder and your other hand at the bottom of the scapula. Now lift the shoulder up and massage underneath the scapula, moving up toward the top. Repeat on the other side. This scapula release is appropriate if the upper thoracic vertebrae are sore.

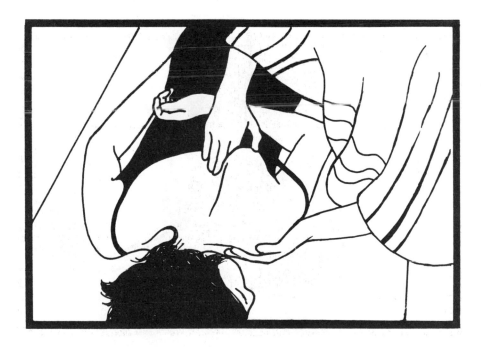

5. Period Pump

This move relieves tension in the hips, thighs and lower back and is great for relieving menstrual difficulties. Move your client's thigh to a 45 degree angle. With your right hand hold the ankle and bring the foot down to the buttocks. Place your left hand over the sacrum. Repeat this pump 15 times, then switch to the other leg.

6. Coccyx Sweep

Place your right hand, palm up, over the coccyx while your left hand slowly brushes down the spine and off the torso. This is a way of releasing all the energy you have brought to the surface.

You may also want to do the chakra balancing exercise at this point (see pages 91–93).

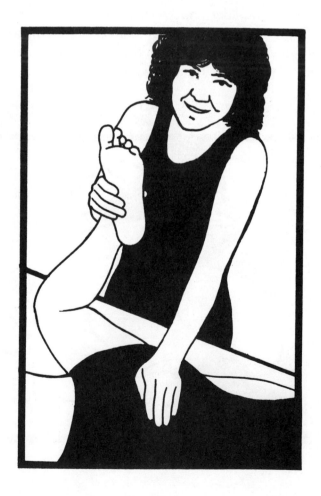

THE HIPS

The hips represent the neutral pole because they are located at the middle of the body. All the energies of the first and second chakras are housed here. Quite often energy collects at the hips from all the impulses that pass downward from the head and upward from the feet. The hips are the home of the *sacrum*, which according to Dr. Stone determines the structural balance throughout the physical body. As the hip area is so vital to our well-being, it is imperative that we keep it clear of any obstructions.

The following set of hip stretches will loosen and maintain the proper elasticity of the hips. Be gentle in your interpretation of these manipulations and you will see how well the body reacts to these simple stretches. Relaxed, elastic hips will maintain the equilibrium necessary for longevity.

These stretches are for both sides, so it doesn't matter where you start. You will quickly discover that each body is unique, so the degree of stretch will vary from person to person. Don't ever stretch too far; go to the point of resistance and then back off a bit. This will assure a gentle stimulation, not a painful experience.

TECHNIQUE FOR THE HIPS

1. Hip Rotation

Place one hand under the knee and with the other hand hold the foot. Bend the knee up and rotate the hip ten times in each direction.

2. Leg Pump

Let your client's leg drop off the table and place it at a 45 degree angle to the other leg. Pump the leg ten times, stretching the top and inside of the thigh.

---

3. Knee-to-Chest Stretch

Stand to either side of the table. Place your upward hand under your client's knee, with your lower hand holding the foot. Gently bend the knee and press it into your client's chest, then into the inside and outside torso. Press five times in each position.

4. Opposite Knee-to-Hip Stretch

Raise your client's leg back up on the table and press the sole of their foot to the opposite knee. Move to the side of the torso. Have your client take a deep breath; on the exhale hold their hip and press down on the knee. Repeat three times. Brush off the thigh and gently place the leg down.

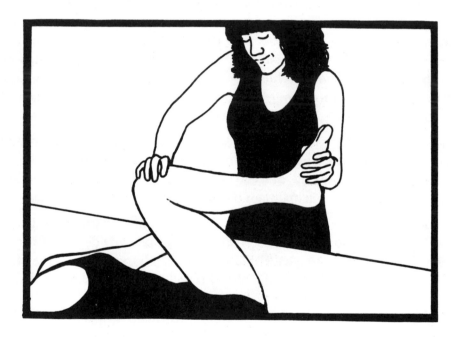

PERINEAL SESSION

The perineal muscles represent the negative pole of the torso. They are the base of the core energy in the torso, and like the base of a pyramid, determine how strong the structure will be. If the foundation is weak, then the structure will surely crumble. Similarly, tension or energy blocks in the perineal muscles cause tension in the entire body, resulting in poor health. However, once the perineal muscles are relaxed, the body's energy currents return to normal, thus maintaining good health.

The impulses of the brain pass through the neck, shoulders, and back to the rest of the body. Sometimes, due to emotional imbalance, stressful situations, or too much mental activity, the outgoing nerve impulses from the brain back up, blocking the incoming impulses. This causes tension that holds the muscles tight. By releasing the perineal muscles, the energy blocks are removed and the currents operate smoothly again. The entire body relaxes in a very deep and nurturing state when the perineal muscles are free from tension. People often go to sleep or enter an altered state of consciousness. This kind of relaxation can be a new experience and the beginning of a greater awareness of who we really are. Any perineal contact will greatly reduce tension in the neck, shoulders and back.

The fire finger is used to make all contacts on the perineal muscles because it is positively charged and the perineal floor is negatively charged, thus creating a perfect polarity contact. All contacts on the perineal muscles are firm, with your fire finger directed toward your client's head. Within ten minutes the perineal muscles should relax and become soft. When this occurs increase your pressure, always keeping a firm contact. Stay in touch with your client and keep the pressure on the contact spot comfortable.

Often you will feel a lot of heat being released at the contact point, and sometimes a pulse. Both responses indicate a deep release of tension, which is exactly what you want!

PERINEAL CONTACT POINTS

1. Contact A

Contact the perineal muscle under the *symphisis pubis* (pubic bone), to the side, with the right fire finger. The thumb and index finger of the left hand contact the occipital ridge of the skull on either side of the spinal column. Contact A is used for nervousness, thyroid cases, sleeplessness, neck pain, general tension and respiration problems.

2. Contact B

Move your right fire finger back about one inch along the perineal floor. Also, move your left hand down about one inch along the neck. Contact B is good for prostate problems in men and uterine problems in women.

3. Contact C

Move your right fire finger back to either side of the anus. Move your left hand down one inch on the neck. Contact C is good for hemorrhoids, colitis and constipation.

4. Contact D

Move your right hand down to the coccyx, just underneath it or on either side of it. Move your left hand down to the shoulders at the trapezius muscle. This contact will release most shoulder pains caused by emotional stress.

PERINEAL TREATMENT

1. Head Cradle and Skull Traction

2. Foot Session

3. Have your client roll on their left side and place a pillow under their head for comfort. Make perineal Contact C and hold for 10 minutes.

4. Do the Spinal Walk while keeping your contact on the perineal floor.

5. Perineal Sweep

Make contact with the air finger of your left hand at the jaw, shoulder, sternum, navel center, hip, knee and ankle. This move will enable you to relax the entire body: everyone enjoys it!

6. Perineal Rock

Release all contacts. Place your left hand on your client's shoulder and your right hand on their buttocks. Gently rock for three minutes.

7. Have your client roll onto their stomach for opposite shoulder-to-hip rocks.

8. Chakra Balancing

9. Neck Cracker

Have your client slowly turn onto their back. Go to either side of the table and with the thumb of your lower hand find a sore spot in the neck. With your upper hand, slowly turn the head into the sore spot thumb contact. Have your client breathe through the pain. Do the other side.

10. Head Cradle

11. Brush off

LENGTHENING THE

SHORT LEG

Between one and two percent of the general population are born with a misaligned hip, leg, foot or spine that causes one leg to be shorter than the other. However, due to stress, lack of exercise, overactive minds, digestive difficulties and emotional disarray, many individuals have developed imbalances within their body, mind and soul. This usually manifests in many ways, depending upon the individual's circumstances. Many people develop a short leg as part of their physical imbalance. Freeing blocked energy and lengthening the short leg will greatly enhance their well-being on a structural level. They will immediately notice a change in their gait as they walk around after the treatment and will probably feel a lot of relief.

Dr. Stone traced many of the structural energy blocks that occur throughout the body to a misaligned sacrum (see *The Mysterious Sacrum*, by Dr. Stone). The sacrum is that part of the spine called the *lower lumbar region*. It consists of five vertebrae fused together and shaped like a triangle with the apex pointing down. Problems develop when the sacrum becomes tilted to either side, rotated back and forth, or any combination of these conditions. Since all the other vertebrae use the sacrum as their base support, any sacral movement will shift the positioning of the spine. A spinal curvature can result, affecting the entire body. Together with the *ilium*, *ischium* and *pubis*, the sacrum forms the *pelvic girdle*. If the pelvis is moved out of its natural position, the bones of the legs, feet and shoulders and the many muscle groups that attach to those bones will be greatly affected. Tight shoulders, headaches, back pain, leg pain and foot pain are just some of the symptoms of a misaligned sacrum. It is one of the key parts of the body and should always be free of tension.

The following manipulations will release blocked energy on the anterior sacral base and lengthen the short leg. It is a gentle, sophisticated stretch that works 99 percent of the time. There are no vertebrae being forced back into place, so it's painless. Sometimes this manipulation will hold for only one day, but often once is all a person needs. It depends on the individual, their lifestyle and how much they want to improve their condition.

TECHNIQUE TO LENGTHEN THE SHORT LEG

1. Method #1

(You can use this technique at any time during the treatment.)
A. *Have your client lie on their back.*

B. *Measuring.* Place each hand below the ankles, along the achilles tendon. Lift the legs up about 18 inches and rotate them five times in each direction. As you gently put the feet down, release your contact and bring the ankle bones together. Now see if they are even. If one ankle bone is longer than the other, the sacrum is out of balance and they need adjustment. If both ankle bones are even, this manipulation isn't necessary.

C. *Positioning.* Move up to the hips of the long leg. At this point inform your client where the contact will be made. Ask your client to locate a tender or sore spot above the pubic bone on the side of the long leg. Place the thumb of your lower hand over the contact spot. The thumb should lie flat on the contact. Remember, you are on the soft tissue right above the pubic bone, on the long-legged side. If you feel confident enough to locate the tender spot yourself, start with your hand at the navel center and slowly move down to the pubic bone until you reach the contact point. Tell your client what you are doing, so as to dispel any anxiety they might have. Place your other hand under the neck.

D. *Stretching.* Have your client take a deep breath. As they exhale, slowly lift the neck and head upward so the chin makes contact with the upper part of the sternum (breast bone). As you lift the neck, gently push down into the tender area with your thumb. When your client finishes the exhalation, release both contacts. Repeat the stretch for a total of three times.

E. *Checking.* Go back down to the feet and recheck the length of the legs by comparing the ankle bones. The ankle bones should be even, indicating even hips and a balanced sacrum.

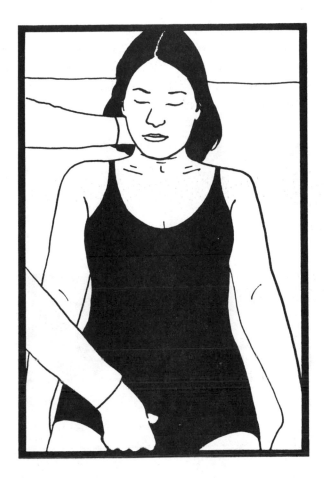

2. Method #2

If the above technique fails to lengthen the short leg, try the following one:

A. *Have your client lie face down.*

B. *Measuring.* Bring the feet together and measure the ankle bones.

C. *Positioning.* Move up to the torso side of the short leg. With your upper hand, locate a sore spot at the top of the *femur* (thigh bone) where it fits into the pelvic girdle. Contact the muscles along either side of the femur and you should find a place that is sensitive to the touch. Place your middle finger on the contact point. Place your other hand under the ankle and gently lift so that the sole of the foot is facing the ceiling.

D. *Stretching*. With the hand holding the ankle, rotate the leg clockwise 15 times. With each rotation, stimulate the contact point on the femur. Then set the leg down and release the femur contact.

E. *Checking.* Check the ankle bones to see if they are even.

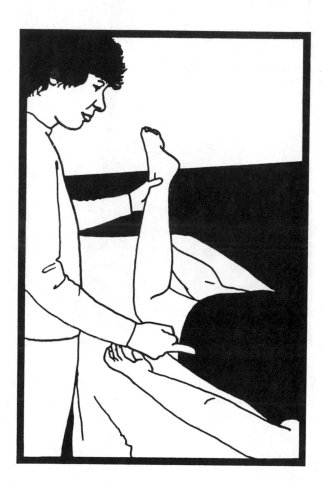

JOINT SESSION

There are millions of people throughout the world seeking relief from painful joints. This can be caused by too much acid accumulating in the joints, causing swelling and low-level pain. The build-up of acid also slows down the entire digestive process.

A change in the kind of foods you eat can help this condition. Avoid all meats, citrus fruits, tomatoes, coffee, sugars, white flour products, salt, tobacco and alcohol. Fresh raw cream and avocados in small quantities act as a lubricating agent and are highly recommended. Your diet should consist of fresh, raw organic fruits and vegetables and grains that are low in acid. The joint session will greatly aid any arthritis condition. All contacts are gentle, so there will be a feeling of nurturance gained from this treatment. Relaxation is the number one result we are aiming for in any session. Only then can your clients heal themselves. Any stress, anxiety or nervous tension will also be neutralized and balanced with this treatment.

The joints are considered neutral, so it doesn't matter what fingers you use while doing this session. As energy travels through the joint, it crisscrosses and reverses itself to the other side. The joints respond together, so both sides will receive benefit from the work done on either side.

DOCTRINE OF SIGNATURES

Things that look alike are alike. The parts of the body that look alike are alike. By using this principle, we can match corresponding parts of the body. Also, by working on one part we can affect its opposite. The following list shows how this principle applies to the body:

Shoulders to hips
Elbows to knees
Wrists to ankles
Hands to feet

Fingers to toes
Chin bone to pubic bone
Arch of foot to spine

TREATMENT FOR THE JOINTS

1. HAve your client lie on the side that does not hurt, with the painful side upright. This will enable your client to be comfortable and to receive the maximum benefit from the treatment. Resting your client's head on a pillow and placing a pillow under their knees will also add to their comfort.

2. Place the thumb of your lower hand a little below the outside ankle point, and the ether and air fingers of your other hand about one inch above the knee. Hold gently for two to three minutes. The knees are the weight-bearing joints of the body and are often sore. It is important to remember that throughout this treatment our contacts are above or below the joint, thus creating an energy field that passes completely through the joint.

3.–7. The lower hand retains contact on the outside ankle point throughout the treatment. The upper hand moves to the hips, then to the shoulder,

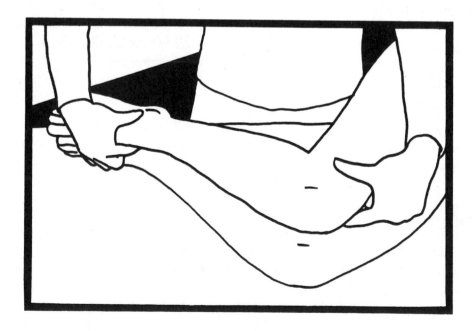

making contact about one inch above the joint. Next move down to the elbow, then to the wrist, and make contact below the joint. Then move to the mid-jaw contact.

8. After you have swept the body, if soreness remains on one particular joint, return to that joint and place the ether and air fingers of both hands about one inch above and below the joint. Hold for two minutes, then create diagonal currents by breaking the contact of one air finger and the ether finger of the other hand. Hold for two minutes, then repeat with the opposite fingers.

Visualize energy going through your fingers in a stream or line; this will speed the healing process. There is really no time limit for any of these contacts. Each situation is different; let your client's need determine what you do.

9. Now, place one hand directly above the joint and the other hand directly below the joint. Hold for five minutes. Quite often you will feel heat, which is a sign of released tension.

A comfrey root poultice applied directly to the joint is very beneficial. Comfrey penetrates deep into the bones and joints, bringing much relief. A grated ginger poultice applied overnight will keep the joint warm and speed the healing process.

THE GENERAL SESSION

Ideally, when all the wireless currents of the body are working in harmony there is good health. The general session is a wonderful way to balance all the body's different energies. It works directly on the three major poles, the head or positive pole, the feet or negative pole and the hips or neutral pole. If one or more of these poles are out of tune, pain and disease will eventually occur. Since this session works on the entire body, any specific ailment your client has should be relieved to some degree. Your client's willingness to relax and let things go will largely affect the results. People respond well to this session and enjoy the feeling of peace it brings.

It is to your advantage to follow this session step by step as indicated at first. After you have mastered the form, feel free to change the sequence of any of the manipulations to suit your own creativity. The form is only as good as the individual using it. Remember, there is no right or wrong way in Polarity Therapy. It's up to you as a practitioner to stay in God's flow and be ready, willing and able to adjust your treatment to suit the needs of the people who come to you. So be open and listen to the inner voice that guides and protects you. It is not necessary to use every manipulation we have learned up to now—use only the ones you feel most comfortable with.

The general session consists of:

1. Three Head Cradles
2. Light neck rub
3. Alternate Shoulder Rock*
4. Five-Pointed Star
5. Foot session
6. Hip session
7. Arms and hands
8. Back session
9. Chakra Balancing
10. Head Cradle
11. Sitting your client up and brushing off
12. Big hug

*Stand at the head of the table, placing a hand on each shoulder. Alternately push each shoulder toward the feet for 30 seconds, then pause for 30 seconds. Repeat three times.

DIAGNOSTIC SIGNS

Reactions take place on many levels during a treatment. The following examples will help you, as a practitioner, understand what is happening, while it is happening.

1. The Fire Element has been activated if your client suddenly gets hungry. Most likely, spots along the digestive tract were activated and the stomach emptied out.

2. The Water Element has been activated when any moisture forms. If sweating is intense, many toxins can be eliminated.

3. The Air Element has been balanced when yawning, sighing or deep breathing occurs. A healthy groan is indicative of Air releases throughout the muscular system.

4. Large earlobes indicate that your client has an excellent vital energy reserve and can fight off illness easier than other people.

5. The Mound of Venus, or soft part of the thumb, is another indicator of a vital energy reserve, as well as the firmness of the buttocks. (See Chart #7, page 108.)

6. The three main lines in the palms of the hands represent the three elements of Air, Fire and Water. The first line, located under the mounds of the fingers, expresses the Fire energy. The clarity, depth, course and length of this line indicate how the body is manifesting the Fire Element. Ovals or cross lines are viewed as energy blocks which limit its expression and interrupt its flow. The Fire line is also known as the heart line and expresses the heart's energy.

7. The head, with the brain and the nervous system, manifests in the Air principle. It is the mind principle that circulates as Air in the blood. In

the palm, the second line expresses the Air quality. It is also called the head line, the home of our thoughts. The appearance of this line tells the story of the Air Element in the body.

8. The Water line originates with the head line and swings in an arc around the Mound of Venus. It reflects the Water Element.

Together, these small diagnostic signs can tell you a lot about your clients and help you to assist them in ways that are most beneficial to them.

EXERCISE

Of all the many wonderful tools we have to maintain good health, exercise does the most to keep the body fit and elastic. When the body is clear and unobstructed, the mind operates more efficiently. And when the mind is ready, man can unite permanently with God. We have many goals we want to accomplish in this life, but these are illusory. Our only true purpose is to achieve union with God through whatever means are available to us. Exercising can be the beginning, for some of us, of that divine quest.

POLAR ENERGETICS

Polar Energetics is a wonderful system of exercise devised by Dr. Randolph Stone. This system of stretching helps you maintain your center and keep your body ready for whatever action your karma dictates.

A daily routine of exercise becomes easier if you set up a specific time and place to practice it in a ritualistic way. The room should be well ventilated and full of sunlight. Loose clothes are recommended, and a carpet or mat should be laid down on the floor. Any incense or candle ceremony with a prayer for good health will enhance the routine. You can offer your aches and pains to the Creator, knowing His love will cure all.

1. Squat

Polar Energetics is based on the posture known as the Squat. What is it about the Squat that makes it so dynamic? In order for the body to properly assimilate all the energy it receives daily, its eliminative function must be in proper working order. Once the body can eliminate wastes easily, it is ready to absorb new stimuli. However, if this eliminative or downward flow is clogged (much the same as a sewer gets backed up), elimination will be stopped and all the circuits will short out, resulting in poor health and disease. The internal downward energy current is governed by the Air principle in the body. Its electrical field is composed of: chest (positive pole) colon (neutral pole) and calves (negative pole). The key is to activate all three poles of this energy field at the same time. This will clear the circuit, freeing any obstructions, whether solid, liquid or gas, to pass on through.

Squatting provides this service to the body. It is so simple that society has completely overlooked its importance in maintaining good health. Just a few minutes daily will keep your muscles and joints elastic and relieve unwanted accumulations of gas.

Stand erect, feet about eighteen inches apart. Take a deep breath and on the exhalation slowly bend your knees until you are down as far as you can go. This will vary greatly from person to person; whatever degree of the Squat you reach is fine—do not strain. If you are having difficulty in going directly down, wiggle from side to side as you begin your descent. Ideally, your feet should be flat on the floor. If this is too difficult and you find yourself on your toes, place a pillow under your heels or wear shoes; this will help your balance and ease the strain on your legs and back. There should be room behind you in case you lose your balance and roll backwards. Your armpits should be directly above your knees with your hands extending out. The posture is now complete.

If you can get into the Squat but have difficulty staying there, hold onto a doorknob or post until the position becomes easier. Do not strain under any circumstances. That would defeat all the good the Squat accomplishes. You are not in competition with anyone, so it doesn't matter where you are when you begin. Improvement will come as you continue. Be patient—there is no fast way!

To start, this position should be held for three minutes a day, with a gradual increase as time goes by. If you feel discomfort in your ankles, calves, thighs, hips, back and neck while you are squatting, this is an indication of where you need to increase your strength.

Once you are in the Squat, the next action is to bounce up and down. This shifts the weight to different muscles. Then move in a circular motion and from side to side. You will be working with many different groups of muscles as you change your position in the Squat.

The easiest way to come out of the Squat is to place both hands on the floor in front of you, shift your weight onto them and slowly stand up, straightening out your head at the very end.

The next variation of the Squat provides a wonderful stretch for your hips. Stand erect with your feet about eighteen inches apart. Slowly go down into the Squat position, with your elbows inside your knees. Now, gently push your knees outward with your elbows. This really works on the hips and lower back and is a great aid in maintaining elasticity in the body.

2. Ha-Frog

The Ha-Frog begins in the Squat position, with your hands over your knees. Slowly raise up into a half-seated position, go back down into the Squat, then use your momentum to bounce back up into the half-seated position. When you reach the Squat position, let out a deep "ha" sound from your navel center. This helps activate the fire energy from within. Start with 15 Ha-Frogs in a continuous motion.

3. Woodchopper

Stand erect with your feet about eighteen inches apart. Reach straight up with joined hands. Bend slightly backward and as you come forward, let your hands swing between your legs, much as you would chop a piece

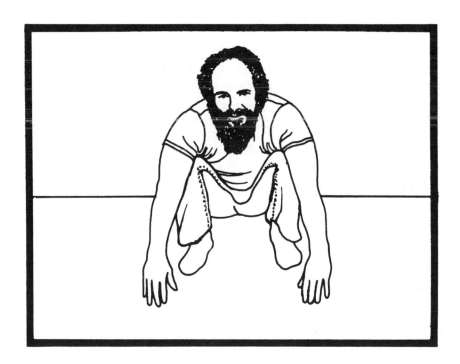

of wood with an axe. Then let your momentum carry you back up to the starting position. As your hands swing between your legs, emitting the "ha" sound will help activate the fire element. Start with 15 Woodchoppers, slowly increasing to about 25.

Both the Ha-Frog and the Woodchopper work with the Fire Element, producing heat and increasing blood circulation. They will increase your energy level, especially if you feel sluggish, depressed or stuck and can't seem to get moving. Your digestion will benefit and your general health will improve once the Fire pattern of your body is functioning well. These exercises increase the action in your cardiovascular system and give the heart a nice short workout.

4. Cliff-Hanger

Stand erect with your back against the edge of a waist-high table. Place your hands, palms open, on the edge of the table. Take a deep breath, and on the exhalation slowly move down into the squat position, placing most of your weight on your brachial plexus. Stay down for about 30 seconds and then slowly come up. As you descend, chanting "OM" will enhance the inward release of stuck energy.

To get the maximum stretch from the Cliff-Hanger, once you are down in the Squat extend your feet straight out so you can wiggle your hips from side to side. All your body weight will be supported by your upper thoracic cavity, which will be receiving a maximum stretch. This will help to clear the chest cavity of blocked energy that could eventually lead to a serious ailment.

This exercise moves energy that has slowed down and remains in deeply blocked patterns throughout the body. As you break through those patterns, the Water Element, which controls the foundation of your body, comes back into balance. This exercise will relieve any stiffness you may find at the brachial plexus or between the shoulder blades.

5. Pyramid

Stand with your feet about eighteen inches apart and the palms of your hands on your knees. Have your elbows locked and bring your shoulders up to your ears: this is the Pyramid Position. Keep your rear down as far as it will go and bounce up and down gently for a few minutes. Then drop your left shoulder toward the center; look over your left shoulder as far as you can and hold for about 15 seconds. Then slowly turn your head over the other shoulder and hold for 15 seconds. Now bring your shoulder back up and repeat this technique for the other shoulder. In the beginning, do this exercise three times. It provides a wonderful stretch for the spine and neck.

6. Spinal Rock

Sit on the floor, placing your hands behind your thighs. Now gently rock back and forth, flexing and stretching the whole back, especially the spine. This will help many back difficulties.

7. Scissor Kicks

Lie on your stomach and bend your legs at the knees. Now swing your feet from side to side, criss-crossing in the middle. Place the emphasis on the outward kick for maximum results. This stretches the hips and activates the cerebrospinal fluid that travels from the sacrum to the brain, relieving sinus discomfort from colds or allergies. It takes about five minutes to be effective.

8. Corpse Position

Lie down on your back with your palms facing up; relax and melt into the floor. This is a wonderful position in which to finish your routine. It promotes deep relaxation and gives the body a chance to integrate all the stretches.

PREGNANCY

Being pregnant can be a wonderful time. When a soul decides to come down from the ethers into human form, it is a very special event. Quite often we think we have complete control of this process, not realizing the soul's part in the drama. After being pregnant and feeling your baby grow inside your belly for nine months, then holding it after it slides out, you begin to understand the beauty of divine creation. Through this experience, you can touch and feel the sacredness of life. Because it is such a holy occasion, the more you prepare yourself and the less you interfere with nature, the easier the whole birth process will be.

AVOIDING TOXINS

One of the main concerns during pregnancy is to avoid all toxins whenever possible and to keep body, mind and spirit in harmony so that the baby can grow and develop at its own pace. Toxins come in many shapes and forms. Some of the major toxins to be avoided are: alcohol, sugar, drugs—including aspirin, antibiotics, marijuana, caffeine, preservatives in food and the lead fumes from filling up your car at the gas station. Even hair permanents contain many chemicals that can be absorbed by the scalp and should be avoided. Wearing high-heeled shoes creates stress on the back and hips; sitting too long in cars has the same effect.

The fetus is affected by any quick eliminating diet, so fasting should be avoided because it puts too much stress on the fetus. As a rule, saunas and hot tubs should be avoided during pregnancy unless the expectant mom has been using them for a while and is careful not to stay too long or keep the temperature too high.

Morning sickness can mean too much hydrochloric acid in the stomach and there are many different types of home remedies that can help: peppermint or chamomile tea, brewer's yeast in a smoothie, eating a cracker or a slice of bread upon rising, or drinking lime juice and water. Vitamin B6 will also help. I personally feel that morning sickness is caused by the mother purifying herself so that her fetus can grow in a clean environment. Chanting and meditation can raise your vibration and help with morning sickness.

HELPFUL HINTS FOR PREGNANT MOTHERS

There are many things recommended as being helpful during pregnancy. Relaxation is perhaps the most important thing; if you are relaxed, everything will go well. Any time you spend being quiet will be beneficial. Meditation and chanting are wonderful tools to call upon God and ease the mind of any worries and fears. Any anxiousness should be avoided.

Simple stretching is helpful. Hatha Yoga, Tai-Chi Chuan and Polar Energetics offer different systems of stretching and breathing that aid in total body awareness and relaxation. Long brisk walks are highly recommended. My wife and I went for long walks along the beach, finding that the negative ions from the ocean cleansed and helped to center us. Squatting is also especially helpful. After birthing Daniel, my wife said that the one thing she should have practiced more to help prepare for the birth was squatting. It is the position that many women use during labor and birth. Having an elastic pelvis makes it much easier, and that is what squatting does.

Swimming gives the body an excellent cardiovascular exercise that is safe and beneficial.

Before birth, it is possible to communicate with your baby by talking to it and rubbing your belly with almond oil. Most babies in the belly enjoy being pampered. Sometimes babies communicate through dreams or meditations, so tune in to your psychic awareness.

Nipple rubs with almond oil and a loofa sponge scrub will toughen the nipples in preparation for breastfeeding. Oil rubs will also help to prevent stretch marks on the belly, thighs and buttocks.

The fetus stores enough iron to last it for six months after birth. So expectant moms must watch what they consume to keep their level of iron high. Floridex, a West German liquid made of concentrated natural fruit juices such as red grapes, blackberries, cherries, pears, yeast and honey, will raise your iron level immediately, restoring the body's proper level of iron within a week. It is also good for expectant papas with low energy. We used this throughout our pregnancy with great results. Calcium is another mineral that the fetus needs for growth, so a calcium supplement is also recommended. Don't take iron and calcium together because they can bind together and not assimilate properly. Wait four to six hours—take one in the morning, the other in the afternoon.

What you eat is tremendously important during pregnancy. A balanced diet of cooked grains, vegetables, fresh fruits and fruit juices, nuts, tofu and the proper supplements are recommended. Raspberry leaf tea is really soothing and contains a lot of iron. Peppermint and chamomile tea can help with digestion.

There may be excess mucus in the nose or vagina; this is a normal occurrence. The body's level of fluids and hormones has been altered, so understand that this excess mucus is just nature working—and trust in her wisdom.

Prenatal classes can teach you many breathing and nutritional guidelines. Find a good midwife or doctor—one you feel comfortable with—and let them guide you through your process. The nesting urge will help you create a place where time just passes by and you can enjoy yourself during this wonderful period of your life.

PREGNANCY SESSION

1. Head Cradle, Skull Traction and Forehead Spread

2. Alternate Shoulder Rock

3. Tummy Rock

4. Opposite Shoulder-to-Opposite Hip Rock

5. Clavicle Rock

With your upper hand, ether and air fingers, make contact on either side of the mid-clavicle bone. Place the thumb of your lower hand below the sternum with fingers overlapping the chest. Rock outward while your thumb moves down along the rib cage. Repeat three times.

6. Foot Session

Omit any ankle work, because it reflexes to the hips, and by stirring up this energy field you could create an adverse effect on the fetus.

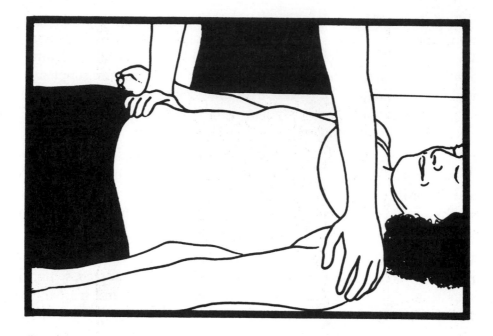

Quite often a pregnant woman has a lot of back and leg pain, so she won't be able to lie on her back for a long period of time. By now she should be ready to slowly move to either side. Then place a pillow under her top leg for comfort. Be sensitive to her needs and have her move as soon as any discomfort appears.

7. Spinal Walk

8. Shoulder-to-Hip Points

Find sore spots at both ends and link them together.

9. Public Bone-to-Orbital Ridge Contact

Have your client turn on her back. Locate any sore spots in front of the pubic bone with your lower hand. Create a diagonal current from one side of the pubic bone to the opposite side of the orbital ridge by the eye. Alternate contacts, then create a new diagonal current. Now move to the mid-pubic bone and mid-chin contact. All above contacts should be held gently.

10. Windshield Wipers

Place your hands on the outside of your client's feet. "Wipe" your hands toward the right, then the left. Brush off.

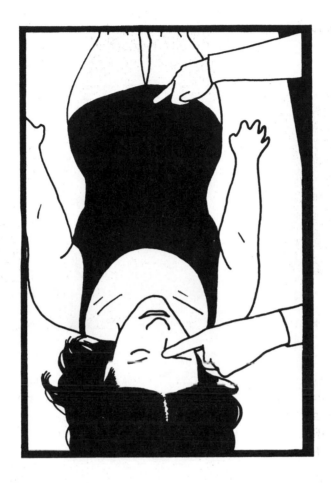

ABOUT FEVER

Fever occurs when the body's temperature rises above its normal range of from 97 to 100 degrees Fahrenheit. Your temperature remains constant regardless of external conditions because your body is always working internally: the diaphragm is expanding and contracting, the chemical action of digestion and assimilation are creating warmth while they do their work. As the work load increases, the amount of heat increases as well. When a fever suddenly appears, your body is working at an accelerated internal pace. Any accumulation of waste material in the blood, tissues and internal organs causes the body to speed up its internal process in an effort to rid itself of these wastes.

Because your body works so silently, you may forget to pay attention to it and pollute it until it has had enough. A fever usually occurs at this point. If you don't change the oil in your car, its performance will decrease and eventually it may overheat. Likewise, if your body doesn't burn off all its accumulated rubbish, it will remain clogged and disease will set in.

Fever is the body's way of cleaning house; we shouldn't interfere with it as long as the fever stays below 105 degrees. Fevers of 105 degrees or more affect the nervous system and can cause damage. However, a fever controlled by keeping the skin cool will usually burn off a disease without any adverse effect. Fever is really our way of healing ourselves, and as long as it's allowed to run its course we'll feel much improved after it subsides, regardless of the disease.

Dehydration can result from the loss of liquids due to sweating, so make sure the person with the fever receives plenty of liquids in the form of freshly squeezed fruit juices. However, consuming any kind of food during a fever can be a mistake because the body's energy is diverted to digesting the food instead of eliminating the toxins. The old adage about "starving a fever" is essentially good advice.

H O M E   A N D   H E R B A L

R E M E D I E S   F O R

C O M M O N   A I L M E N T S

SORE THROAT

1. Salt-water Gargle

One of the quickest, easiest and least expensive remedies for a sore or hoarse throat is a salt-water gargle. Add one teaspoon of salt to a glass of warm water and gargle. This gargle will bring instant relief and can be used three to five times a day. Note: A sore throat is usually the first sign of a cold or flu. Fasting or eating lightly is recommended in order to allow the body to use its energy to fight the cold.

2. Vitamin C

Dissolving a vitamin C tablet in your mouth will help bring relief from a sore throat. Your body uses a lot of vitamin C while defending itself against a cold or flu. You can increase your daily intake to about 2000 mg. a day at the very first sign of a cold. After your symptoms disappear, reduce the vitamin C level gradually, instead of suddenly stopping it, or your reserve supply will be drained.

3. Special Tea

Lemon, honey and cayenne pepper tea is also wonderful for a cold. Add a cup of hot water to the fresh juice of one lemon. Also add a teaspoon of raw honey and a pinch of cayenne pepper. Drink three to five cups a day as soon as you notice a cold coming on. This tea will bring quick relief: the honey will coat and soothe your throat, the lemon will increase your vitamin C level and the cayenne pepper will increase your blood circulation, giving your entire system a boost.

4. Garlic

Garlic has been used by many cultures for treating different illnesses. It is a very powerful natural antibiotic: chewing one or two cloves a day will knock out any cold or flu. Don't worry about the garlic breath that may result; it's a small price to pay for getting well. Chewing on a small piece of fresh parsley will take away your garlic breath. Raw garlic is very hot when eaten, so you can drink water to help lessen the burning sensation. If garlic is too strong for you to eat raw, try cutting it into small pieces and putting it in your shoes. The garlic will be absorbed through your feet into your system within 30 minutes. If you don't wear shoes, try taking garlic oil capsules. They are easy to take, don't burn your mouth and leave no odor. The point is to get garlic into your system. After your sickness is over, remember to eat some food that contains acidophilus to reintroduce the friendly bacteria that your intestines need for proper digestion. Garlic will destroy *all* intestinal bacteria, both good and bad, so it's important to put some back after you take any antibiotic.

SORE MUSCLES

1. Tiger Balm

Tiger Balm is a salve which has been developed in China. Its active ingredients are camphor, menthol, cajeput oil and clove oil. It stimulates circulation by inducing heat in the congested area. Tiger Balm is for external use only and can be applied as often as necessary to muscle spasms, congestion or joint stiffness. My family and friends have used this product for many years. It is part of our herbal first-aid kit and we take it wherever we go.

2. Ginger Wrap

Ginger is a wonderful and effective stimulant. It increases circulation and produces warmth when applied externally. To use, grate about three ounces of fresh ginger and apply directly over the painful joint or muscle spasm. Wrap it with a cotton cloth until it is completely covered and leave it on overnight. In about 30 minutes you will feel a lot of heat and you may think that blisters are developing. But don't worry—no blisters will form. If the heat is too intense, and the ginger can't be left on overnight, leave it on for as long as possible. The ginger wrap will bring great relief. If fresh ginger is not available, make a paste from dried ginger by adding a little water to it and use it as you would fresh ginger.

3. Muscle Liniment

This liniment is an excellent remedy for aching muscles and can be used as a disinfectant to clean cuts and bruises as well. Ingredients: 1 quart jar, 1 oz. of goldenseal powder, 1 oz. of myrrh powder, 1/2 oz. of cayenne pepper powder, 1 pint of rubbing alcohol. Combine all the ingredients in the jar, seal it and set it aside in a dark, cool place. Shake it once a day for two weeks, then strain it through cheesecloth into a dark glass container and label it. Use freely on any cuts, scrapes, bruises or muscle spasms.

4. Arnica Oil

Arnica oil is a homeopathic remedy that can be used externally for all sore or spastic muscles and joints. It reduces the pain level and tenderness associated with aching muscles and joints and can be applied directly to the painful area as often as necessary.

BURNS

1. Ice

Ice is one of the best remedies for burns. When applied immediately to the burn, it brings instant relief by cooling and soothing. Ice or ice water can be kept directly on the burn indefinitely. If the burn is serious, consult a physican as soon as possible.

2. Aloe Vera

The aloe vera plant has been used for centuries to soothe and relieve pain from burns. Simply cut a leaf from the plant, remove the prickly edges and slice the leaf, exposing its jelly-like inner pulp. This pulp can be applied directly to any burn and will instantaneously reduce pain and irritation. Keep an aloe vera plant around the house and it will be readily available when you need it.

BOILS AND PIMPLES

1. Natural Clay

Natural clay has tremendous drawing power and has been successfully used by many people to bring boils and pimples to the surface for proper elimination. Add a little water to a teaspoon of clay and form a paste. Cover the boil or pimple with the clay paste. As it dries, you may experience your skin pulling together, but that is the natural reaction, so don't worry about it. Leave the clay on overnight and the condition should be improved by morning. Clay can also be used on any rash, especially poison oak or poison ivy, to stop itching and dry it up. Clay is also effective on insect bites.

2. Beets

Dr. Stone says that grated raw beets applied directly to a boil with a cotton cloth and left on overnight will reduce the boil to almost nothing by morning. I have used this remedy myself with fantastic results and I strongly recommend it.

HEADACHE

According to Dr. Stone, many headaches are caused by poor digestion and assimilation of food, which results in the production of gas. As the gas moves upward to escape, it lodges in the muscles, bones, organs, etc. By watching your diet you may be able to change your headache pattern.

1. Tiger Balm

Tiger Balm rubbed on the temples or forehead sometimes brings relief from headaches. It is a stimulant and brings fresh blood to the area, breaking through the congestion.

2. Baths

Filling up the tub with hot water and sitting on the edge with your feet in the water is an excellent remedy for any headache. It draws the blocked energy down from your head to your feet and reconnects the long energy currents of the body. Try it.

3. Foot Rub

A vigorous foot massage will sometimes bring relief from headaches. The feet have reflex points to places all over the body and a good massage can get the energy moving again.

SPECIAL HOME REMEDIES

The following home remedies have been compiled from notes taken during a workshop with Pierre Pennetier in November 1981, Santa Cruz, California:

1. Parsley tea can relieve indigestion and help restore proper breathing. It is also good for kidney trouble.

2. Coffee and parsley are diuretics and stimulate the kidneys.

3. Parsley tea can be an abortive, so is not recommended during pregnancy.

4. To help dissolve and remove any stone in the system, combine four tablespoons of olive oil and two tablespoons of lemon juice with fresh parsley tea made from at least five stems of parsley.

5. For an ear infection, crush three garlic cloves and add to olive oil in an amber container. After two weeks use this mixture with a Q-tip in the affected ear.

6. Garlic soup is good for worms in the intestines.

7. Garlic eases hardening of the arteries, capillaries and veins, and restores their elasticity.

MISCELLANEOUS REMEDIES

1. To counteract exposure to radiation, drink the Liver Flush (see page 70) daily for one month.

2. To remove heavy metal or lead poisoning, alternate daily baths of one cup Clorox bleach to a full bath with one pound of sea salt plus one pound of baking soda to a full bath. Alternate for ten days.

3. To neutralize chemical spraying of fruits and vegetables, add one tablespoon of Clorox bleach to a gallon of water and soak the food for 30 minutes.

4. For lower back pain, draw a warm bath and add a pot of strained chamomile tea.

5. Squatting is good for relieving any pain in the legs.

6. For menstrual cramps, pull on your tongue.

7. To help relieve sciatica, cut back on protein consumption, including cheese, soy beans, yogurt and meat.

8. To stop diarrhea, mash a raw apple and add a little cinnamon to it.

9. For dysentery, add blackberry juice to a mashed raw apple and cinnamon.

10. For constipation, combine two ounces of olive oil with four ounces of fresh lemon juice and take three times a day.

11. Soak all dried fruits, nuts and seeds to bring back the life-force energy before you eat them.

12. Black pepper is good for a cold or flu.

13. Honey is a mild laxative.

14. Fennel tea is good for producing mother's milk.

15. Lemon juice eyewash is good for glaucoma or cataracts. (One part lemon juice to seven parts water.)

16. Rub lemon peel on your face to keep the skin smooth.

17. Any bitter herb tea, such as one made from artichoke leaves, will help cleanse the liver.

18. For any foot infection, take a foot bath with the tea of rosemary, thyme, sage and clove.

19. Celery juice is good for the nerves.

20. Alternate hot and cold showers are good for circulation.

21. For an ulcer, mix the juice of cabbage, celery, carrot and lemon together with cayenne pepper and drink twice a day.

22. Apply ice to a sprained ankle.

23. Saliva is good on any fresh cut.

24. For rheumatism or arthritis, take a foot bath with stinging nettle tea or goat's milk.

25. Burdock and dandelion tea are excellent blood purifiers.

26. For morning sickness or nausea, take an orange leaves tea bath.

27. Dandelion root tea is good for plantar's warts.

28. Cayenne pepper sprinkled in your shoes will keep you warm and help your circulation.

29. Juniper berry tea is good for cramps; drink daily for one week.

QUIETING THE MIND

Through the experience of life, you eventually discover your own consciousness and your true relationship to the cosmos. As you wander down the road of life, you learn and experience many useful things. The reality of the physical world has a way of jumping up at you and demanding that you meet certain criteria for survival. For many of us the battle to maintain a certain material standard overshadows our true purpose in life—to experience peace, happiness and union with God.

MEDITATION

Meditation is a mental technique specifically designed to help you reach the goal of inner peace. It accomplishes this by stopping the continuous flow of thoughts generated day and night by your overactive mind. When your mind is always filled there's no room to receive divine energy from the universe. This concept is very simple, yet it is often overlooked as we seek complex solutions to the complex situations we have created. Life is not that complex, but through our fears, worry and anxiety we have become our own worst enemy by preventing the love energy from flowing freely among us. Our society has accomplished this by setting certain social standards that breed fear and don't allow for the expression of love openly. For example, in many parts of our country it is illegal or unacceptable for a mother to breastfeed her infant in public. I can't think of a more loving gesture than breastfeeding, yet it is met with so much negativity by the public. Another example is to walk down the busy street of a large city like New York and say hello to the people you pass. The reaction is unbelievable. Most people won't respond or acknowledge you at all. Others will just give you an angry or bewildered look. Once a middle-aged woman stopped and said to me in an aggressive tone, "I don't know you—so why are you saying hello to me?" You wouldn't think that merely saying hello to your fellow human beings would be met with so much hostility—yet it happens every day. The point is, we need to slow down and take the time to share love before we close down completely and stop expressing it entirely. Being afraid to express the love we feel inside us leads to feelings of unfulfillment. By encouraging toughness and selfishness we don't allow the soft, gentle side of our nature to emerge.

Meditation is the cosmic link between humans and the Creator. The person who continuously practices meditation will slowly be able to wipe clean the slate of negative thought patterns and refill the empty space with love. Once the love connection with the universe is established, life becomes easier and the obstacles that once seemed to threaten us become easier to deal with.

ALTERNATIVE NOSTRIL BREATHING

For thousands of years saints and sages from the Himalayan Mountains of India have helped the peoples of the world by sharing simple meditation techniques that have been scientifically proven to be effective. One such breathing technique is called *alternative nostril breathing*. Alternative nostril breathing is one of the most powerful breathing techniques because it works on many different levels of growth at the same time.

Alternative nostril breathing immediately quiets the mind and is a great way to prepare yourself for meditation. It can stop an anxiety attack, relieve a headache, calm the emotions and soothe any anger that temporarily takes over. It reconnects the mind to the soul and recharges the spirit and is one of the best ways to deal with the stress caused by our fast-paced lives. Become familiar with the technique, so it will be available to you whenever you need it.

Sit comfortably in a chair or crosslegged on the floor. Close your eyes and relax. Inhale slowly through both nostrils, then close off your right nostril with the right thumb of your right hand. Exhale completely through your left nostril. Now inhale through your left nostril, close it off with your right little finger and exhale through your right nostril. Inhale through your right nostril, close it off with your right thumb and exhale through your left nostril. Repeat the technique ten times, twice a day—once in the morning and again in the evening. Slowly work on increasing to 20 rounds. This is one of the best ways to breathe: you receive many benefits on many levels. Alternate nostril breathing transmits the life force from the ethers into the body at an accelerated pace. You receive seven times more oxygen using this technique than through normal breathing. It cleanses the two major currents that run along either side of the spine called *Ida* and *Pingala*. These currents are the pathway for the Kundalini energy as it rises from the base of the spine on its journey to the crown chakra.

THE POLARITY

LOVE CIRCLE

The Polarity Love Circle is a beautiful experience. It is a true expression of love facilitated by the gentle touch. Everyone involved will be uplifted, especially the person receiving the love energy.

Have your client lie on their back on a massage table or floor. Those who are suffering on any level will benefit the most from receiving the love energy. The people who are making contact are positioned at different locations around the table. Have one person move down to the client's feet and make contact on the inside ankle point of both feet with their air fingers. Another person holds the head in a Head Cradle. A third person stands on the right side of the table with their left hand on the client's left shoulder and their right hand on the client's right hip. Another person is situated on the left side of the table with their right hand on the client's right shoulder and their left hand on the client's left hip. Another person is on the right side of the table with their left hand on the client's right hip and their right hand on the client's right ankle. Another person is on the left side of the table with their right hand on the client's left hip and their left hand on the client's left ankle. There are now six people making contact with the client.

There is no movement during the Polarity Love Circle. Everyone holds the contacts from five to fifteen minutes. Soft chanting of the mantra "OM" by the people making contact can enhance the experience for everyone. If chanting isn't appropriate, just close your eyes and hold the contact while sending out love energy. The energy will do the work, so trust it. When you break contact, each person should slowly come out of the energy field gently, one by one, starting with the contacts at the feet.

After everyone has broken contact, let the client rest quietly. Usually, within five minutes they will be ready to get up. Ask for feedback and let them talk about their experience. Other people in the circle can also share what they felt. You'll be surprised how well your friends and relatives will respond to this simple but powerful exchange of love energy. You can perform this love circle at family gatherings or with groups of friends to help one another open the doors of love. Good luck.

SONGS TO OPEN

THE HEART

Singing the Lord's name is another pathway many people take in their quest for union with God. By immersing yourself in the constant singing of the Lord's name, your consciousness will eventually assume the quality of oneness with Him. Some chants originate with the American Indians, some with the people of India, some with the Sufis.

The following chants and songs are designed to help you forget about yourself, turn off your mind and tune into God. Let all your chanting come from your heart, and enjoy the peace it brings!

DEFINITIONS OF SANSKRIT WORDS IN CHANTS AND SONGS

1. Ananda: Peace.
2. Bhagavan: Lord—Vishnu.
3. Bhakti: Devotion to the Lord.
4. Hanuman: Monkey God who is the perfect servant of Lord Rama.
5. Hare: Formal address to Lord God.
6. Hari: Another name for Vishnu.
7. Jai: Glory.
8. Jaya: Victory.
9. Krishna: An incarnation of God.
10. Maha: Great.
11. Om: The holy sound of all cosmic vibration.
12. Rama: An incarnation of Vishnu.
13. Shanti: Peace.
14. Shiva: Deity that presides over the destructive energies of life. Known as the cosmic cleanser.

15. Shri: A title of reverent respect.
16. Sita: Rama's Wife.
17. Vasudeva: He who abides in all things.

CHANTS AND SONGS

1. We all come from God
   And unto God we shall return (2 times)
   Like a stream flowing down
   To the ocean
   Like a ray of light
   Returning to the sun.

2. Blessed am I
   Freedom am I
   I am the infinite
   Within my soul
   I can find no beginning
   I can find no end
   Oh yes I am.

3. Happiness runs in a circular motion
   Life is like a little boat upon the sea
   Everybody is a part of everything anyway
   You can have it all if you let yourself be.

4. Where I sit is holy
   Holy is the land
   Forest, mountain, river
   Listen to the sound
   Great spirit circle all around me.

5. Enna May, Enna May, Ennana mitchie chiow. (2 times)
   Enna mitchie choiw. (4 times)

6. Oh sing my heart sing
   Let my eyes gaze upon thee
   Upon my Lord (2 times)
   Hare Ram, Hare Ram, Rama, Rama, Hare, Hare,
   Hare Ram, Hare Ram.

7. The earth, the water, the fire the air,
   Returns, returns, returns, returns (2 times)
   Hey yay, yay, yay, yay, yay, yay, yay,
   Wo, wo, wo, wo, wo, wo, wo. (2 times)

8. Sri Ram, Jai Ram, Jai Jai Ram (4 times)
   Jai Sita Ram, Jai Jai Hanuman (2 times)
   Sri Guru Om Ananda Bhagavan. (2 times)

9. Dear friend, dear friend,
   This I have to say to you
   You have given me your blessings
   I love you, I love you.

10. May the blessings of God
    Rest upon you
    May Her peace abide with you
    May Her presence illuminate your heart
    Now and forever more.

11. We are opening up in sweet surrender
    To the infinite power of the Lord (2 times)
    We are opening, we are opening (2 times)
    We are opening up in sweet surrender
    To the infinite wisdom of our soul (2 times)
    We are opening, we are opening. (2 times)

12. May we all fly like eagles
    Flying so high
    Circle in the universe
    On wings of pure light
    Oh witchie chai o
    Oh way hi o
    Oh witchie chai o
    Oh way hi o.

13. Rama Rama, Rama Rama
    Rama Rama, Mangalam (2 times)
    Ramakrishna vasudeva
    Bhakti mukti dhayakam. (2 times)

14. All I ask of you
    Is forever to remember me (2 times)
    As loving you
    Ishg Allah Ma'abud L'illah. (2 times)

15. Om Shanti, Om Shanti. (repeat over and over)

BIBLIOGRAPHY

CHAKRAS AND KUNDALINI

Gunther, Bernard. *Energy Ecstasy*. N. Hollywood, CA: Newcastle, 1983.
Madhusudandasji, Dhyan Yogi Shri. *Shakti: Hidden Treasure of Power*. Clayton, CA: Dhyan Yoga Centers, 1980.
Rhada, Swami Sivananda. *Kundalini: Yoga for the West*. Boulder, CO: Shambhala, 1981.

DIET

Airola, Paavo. *Are You Confused?* Phoenix: Health Plus, 1971.
Ballentine, Rudolph. *Diet and Nutrition*. Honesdale, PA: Himalayan International Institute, 1978.
Kushi, Michio. *The Book of Macrobiotics*. Scranton, PA: Harper & Row, 1977.
Nelson, Dennis. *Food Combining Simplified*. Santa Cruz, CA: The Plan, 1985.
Stone, Randolph. *Health-Building*. Reno, NV: CRCS Publishers, 1963.

HATHA YOGA AND POLAR ENERGETICS

Devananda, Vishnu. *The Complete Illustrated Book of Yoga*. NY: Washington Square Press, 1972.
Satchidananda, Swami. *Integral Yoga*. NY: Holt, Rinehart & Winston, 1970.
Stone, Randolph. *Easy Stretching Postures*. Reno, NV: CRCS Publishers, 1954.

MANTRAS

Keshavadas, Satguru Sant. *Healing Techniques of the Holy East.* Oakland, CA: Vishwa Dharma Publishers, 1980.

Madhusudandasji, Dhyan Yogi Shri. *Brahmanad: Mantra, Sound and Power.* Clayton, CA: Dhyan Yoga Centers, 1979.

Radha, Swami Sivananda. *Mantras: Words of Power.* Porthill, ID: Timeless Books, 1980.

PREGNANCY

Airola, Paavo. *Every Woman's Book.* Phoenix: Health Plus, 1979.

Gardner, Joy. *Healing the Family.* NY: Bantam Books, 1982.

Gaskin, Ina May. *Spiritual Midwifery.* Summertown, TN: Book Publishing Co., 1978.

Glas, Norbert. *Conception, Birth and Early Childhood.* Spring Valley, NY: Anthroposophic Publishers, 1983.

Kitzinger, Sheila. *The Experience of Childbirth.* NY: Penguin Books, 1972.

Leboyer, Frederick. *Birth Without Violence.* NY: Knopf, 1975.

Parvati, Jeannine. *Prenatal Yoga.* Monroe, UT: Freestone Press, 1978.

OTHER POLARITY THERAPY BOOKS

Gordon, Richard. *Your Healing Hands.* Berkeley, CA: Bookpeople, 1978.

Siegel, Alan. *Life Energy.* San Francisco: Polarity Therapy Center, 1983.

OTHER BOOKS BY DR. RANDOLPH STONE

Energy, the Vital Principle in the Healing Art. 1957.
The Mysterious Sacrum. 1954.
The Mystic Bible. 1956.
Polarity Therapy. 1959.
Vitality Balance. 1957.
The Wireless Anatomy of Man. 1953.

To purchase any of Dr. Stone's books, contact CRCS Publishers, P.O. Box 20850, Reno, NV 89515.

MISCELLANEOUS

Anderson, Mary. *Colour Healing.* York Beach, ME: Samuel Weiser, 1975.

Brown, Deena. *American Yoga.* NY: Grove Press, 1980.

Dass, Baba Hari. *Hariakhan Baba—Known, Unknown.* Davis, CA: The Sri Rama Foundation, 1975.

Dass, Ram. *Miracle of Love.* NY: Dutton, 1979.

Lad, Dr. Vasant. *Ayurveda: The Science of Self Healing.* Santa Fe, NM: Lotus Press, 1984.

Muramoto, Naboru. *Healing Ourselves.* NY: Avon, 1973.

Pritikin, Nathan. *The Pritikin Promise.* NY: Pocket Books, 1982.

Rama, Swami. *Living with the Himalayan Masters.* Honesdale, PA: The Himalayan Institute of Yoga, 1978.

Tierra, Michael. *The Way of Herbs.* Santa Cruz, CA: Unity Press, 1980.

Yogananda, Paramahansa. *Man's Eternal Quest.* Los Angeles: Self-Realization Fellowship, 1975.